Professional Responsibili

SERIES EDITOR

June Clark BA MPhil SRN HVCert

In the same Series

Professional Responsibility

Second Edition

MONICA E. BALY BA(Hons) SRN SCM HVCert

Researcher for the Nightingale Fund Council; formerly Regional Officer, Royal College of Nursing and Lecturer and Examiner for the Diploma in Nursing

An HM + M Nursing Publication

JOHN WILEY & SONS

Chichester · New York · Brisbane · Toronto · Singapore

HM + M is an imprint of JOHN WILEY & SONS LTD

Library of Congress Cataloging in Publication Data:
Baly, Monica E. (Monica Eileen)
    Professional responsibility.
    (Topics in community health) (HM + M nursing
publication)
    Rev. ed. of: Professional responsibility in the
community health services. 1975.
    Bibliography: p.
    Includes index.
    1. Community health nursing. 2. Nursing ethics.
3. Nurse practitioners. I. Baly, Monica E. (Monica
Eileen). Professional responsibility in the community
health services. II. Title. III. Series. IV. Series:
HM + M nursing publication.
RT98.B34   1983   610.73′43   83-16770

ISBN 0 471 26284 6 (U.S.)

British Library Cataloguing in Publication Data:
Baly, Monica E.
    Professional responsibility. — 2nd ed. —
    (Topics in community health). — (An HM + M nursing publication)
    1. Social workers — Great Britain
    2. Social workers, Professional ethics
    I. Title   II. Series
    362.1′023   RA485

ISBN 0 471 26284 6

Phototypeset by Dobbie Typesetting Service, Plymouth, Devon.
Printed by Pitman Press Ltd., Bath, Avon.

To the late June Buttimore
and
to Eva who cared for her

Contents

Preface

The first edition of *Professional Responsibility* was designed as a short guide for health workers in the community in matters relating to their professional, legal and moral responsibilities. It was written while the health services were being reorganised — ostensibly to produce a unified and integrated service. The second edition has been written against the background of further reorganisation made necessary by the heavy super-structure created in 1974. However, whatever the failings of the various reorganisations, to a large extent the main aim, that of unification, has been achieved, inasmuch as all health workers — though not social workers — in any one district are employed by the same health authority.

Partly because of this, but largely because the changing health needs of the community have forced a different response which has been reflected in the education of health workers, communications between the hospital and the primary care teams are better. Although still far from perfect, there are closer links between the arms of the service and it is now less appropriate to write a book which deals with the professional, legal and ethical problems of one section as if they were exclusive brethren. Indeed, to do so would run counter to the philosophy that it is one service giving care in a variety of different places. Although the emphasis may be on different facets, professional responsibility is the same in the hospital ward as it is in the doctor's surgery, the school, the workplace or the patient's home, and lack of professional responsibility will have the same effect, and probably spring from the same source. The law is the same for the nurse in hospital as it is in the community, though one group may be more prone to falling foul of its dictates, or more vunerable, than another. Ethics are nothing if they are not about principles, and principles do not change and are the same for the hospital worker as they are for the health worker in the community. The second edition therefore has drawn on wider material and should be of use not only in the community but to all health workers who are concerned with these problems.

In the past seven years the need to think more clearly about professional responsibility and what we mean by it has become more urgent. Firstly, the services are more complicated and involve more workers, which, together with the increasing use of computers makes the problem of confidentiality more difficult. Secondly, the extended role of the nurse and the increasing use of the nursing process means that nurse must think more carefully about accountibility and the responsibility for their own actions. They cannot claim to be the 'independent pre-scribers of care' and not accept responsibility for their prescrip-tion, and for the planning and implementation of their nursing plans. Thirdly, there is, and will continue to be, an increasing proportion of patients who are vunerable and who are likely to tax our moral philosophy to the utmost: these include the very old, those kept alive on machines, the severely mentally and physically handicapped and the immigrant population who have not integrated into the host culture. Lastly, society in general has a greater expectation for care. In 1892, Miss Nightingale in an address to nurses wrote "Primary education has made our patients, especially our new patients, much sharper than they were in observing us and in criticising us". Plus la change plus c'est la même chose.

The material in this book is still largely based on experience gained in helping with problems raised by members of the Royal College of Nursing and trying to solve them together; this has been supplemented by discussions on these matters with the Diploma in Nursing students; human problems have a way of remaining the same.

As with the first edition, this book cannot give easy answers because each problem is separate and unique. It will be something if the book is able to suggest to practitioners the right questions or even alert them to the fact that there are questions to be asked. If answers are suggested, then they are on the plane of generality which it is hoped will make possible their answer to many problems.

Bath
September 1983

MONICA E. BALY

Acknowledgements

Although the second edition of *Professional Responsibility* is virtually a new book my indebtedness remains the same to those who helped with the first edition, particularly to Mrs Betty Newstead without whose counsel and guidance the first edition would not have been attempted, and with whom I so often discussed 'what is the right thing to do'.

I still acknowledge a debt to the late Mrs Norah Mackenzie who first led me to take an interest in moral philosophy and to those various tutors who have helped me since. Also, although he does not know it, to The Rector of Bath Abbey, who is always wise on ethical issues.

In preparing the second edition I have received help from the Royal College of Nursing and particularly to the Western Area Office where I have been allowed access to references and where the officers were always helpful about discussing problems that were relevant to this subject.

My thanks are also due to June Clark, the editor of the series, who first suggested that there was a need for such a book and who helped in identifying the questions that needed to be asked, and to Mr Patrick West, our editor from HM + M days and still happily with us 'to warn, to comfort and command'.

1983   MEB

Translation of the Hippocratic Oath given by Dr. Charles Singer in his *Greek Biology and Greek Medicine* (1932).

"I swear by Apollo the healer, and Aesculapius and Hygeia, and All-heal (Panacea) and all the gods and goddesses . . . that, according to my ability and judgement, I will keep this oath and this stipulation — to reckon him who taught me this Art as dear to me as those who bore me, . . . to look upon his offspring as my own brothers, and to teach them this Art, if they would learn it, without fee or stipulation. By precept, lecture, and all other modes of instruction, I will impart a knowledge of the Art to my own sons, and those of my teacher, and to disciples bound to me by a stipulation and oath according to the Law of Medicine; but to none other. I will follow that system of regimen which, according to my ability and judgement, I consider for the benefit of my patients, and abstain from whatever is deleterious and mischievous. I will give no deadly medicine to any one if asked, nor suggest any such counsel; nor will I aid a woman to procure an abortion. With purity and holiness I will pass my life and practise my Art . . . . Into whatsoever houses I enter, I will go there for the benefit of the sick, and will abstain from every act of mischief and corruption; and above all from seduction . . . . Whatever in my professional practice — or even not it connection with it — I see or hear in the lives of men which ought not to be spoken of abroad, I will not divulge, deeming that on such matters we should be silent. While I keep this Oath unviolated, may it be granted me to enjoy life and the practice of the Art, always respected among men but should I break or violate this Oath, may the reverse be my lot."

Chapter 1

The Hallmarks of a Profession

"It is a measure of the failure of the present National Health Service pay determination arrangements to provide pay which is fair, either absolutely or relatively, that National Health Services workers — doctors, nurses, ambulancemen, administrators, radiographers and electricians — have increasingly felt, and demonstrated, that only traditional industrial action can resolve their grievances."

Improving Industrial Relations in the N.H.S.
A Report by the TUC Health Services Committee, 1981

Whether industrial action can resolve the grievances of workers in the Health Service is a matter of opinion, but it is an undeniable fact that in the last decade the most unlikely groups, including doctors and nurses, have certainly contemplated such action. This is, of course, one indicator of a changing scene, in which, as the TUC document rightly points out, "the distinctions between unions and professional associations becoming blurred".[1] In the light of this change the public could be forgiven if they regard the claim of the professions to special status as an anachronism, and attempts to define professional responsibility as a waste of time. But in spite of an increasingly egalitarian — if not a more equal — society, the proverbial man on the top of the Clapham omnibus would probably agree that life would be poorer if there were not groups whom he instinctively recognises as 'professions'. These he might well identify as people who give a special service to the public which entails a long training, and that such people are motivated by a conviction that the public they serve are entitled to their best endeavours, and that this is something which transcends the usual rules of the market place. He would also probably agree that no one can put a cash price on such things as justice, health, or education, and that society itself must reward such services on a

1

basis that is not only fair when compared with other occupations, but which allows the professional practitioner to pursue further knowledge and to improve his special skills.

What are the Professions?

Broadly speaking the professions are concerned with the services which were once given by the Catholic Church. The early Church had a near monopoly of learning and was responsible for most of the health care, the distribution of welfare, teaching, law making, the training of administrators and, if the Crusaders are included, the upper echelons of the army. With the break-up of feudalism and the growth of the universities this monopoly was gradually weakened and universities began to replace the Church as a training ground for administrators and lawyers. Later, in the sixteenth century, with the growth of the 'new learning', the ideas of the Renaissance and the upheavals of the Reformation, in Protestant countries—and to a lesser extent in Catholic countries—responsibility for public services passed to secular control. Each service developed along a different and pragmatic path. In Elizabethan England the 'welfare' services were largely taken over by the Parish, and the Vestry and Overseers who administered the new Poor Laws. These laws, and the Parish, were concerned with three main groups: the sick poor, those with no work, and the rogues and vagabonds—in other words, the long-term sick and cripples, the unemployed and the miscreants. The Protestant ethic put a heavy emphasis on family responsibility for the individual, whereas the countries of the Counter-reformation tended to continue to favour institutions and religious orders as vehicles for such services as health care, welfare and the teaching of children. This is a point worth remembering because it is the background tradition of a number of our partners in the European Economic Community.

In the eighteenth century society became more complicated and, as the populations grew and wealth increased, philanthropic endeavour began to supplement Parish relief, particularly for groups regarded as 'worthy' such as orphans, or persons hit by sudden misfortune such as crippling. Often spurred on by the zealous preaching of the new non-conformists, in England this period saw the founding of a number of Charity hospitals—the forerunners of the voluntary system which in a later period played such an important role in the development of hospital care.

In the census of 1841 the only acknowledged professions were 'divinity, physics and the law'—physics generally meant university-trained physicians. By 1881 the list had grown to 19 occupations which included such groups as solicitors, surveyors, accountants and the higher Civil Service, but not teachers, except those engaged in higher education. It is not surprising that at this time some people in 'reformed nursing' tried to hitch their waggon to the prevailing professional star and seek registration and the limitation of entry into nursing.

There were a number of reasons for this social change. Firstly, there was the growing complexity of urban life, the demands of the Empire and the increased need for expert services of all kinds. Secondly, in a situation that was largely self-fulfilling, the new wealth produced a growing middle class whose sons, educated at the new public schools, looked for occupations, not in the trade of their forebears, but in public service. Thirdly, there was the demographic change coupled with the problem of entailed estates; younger sons—and much later, daughters—needed to find useful, and socially acceptable, occupations. Nor should the fact be overlooked that the middle classes of the nineteenth century were imbued with religious principles and ideas which they discussed at great length, and that those who had the luxury of choosing an occupation often looked to one that gave service to their fellow men, and in the prevailing ethos thus carried social approval.

The quintessential professional man of the nineteenth century was the independent practitioner whose work was largely unsupervised except occasionally by professional societies or associations of his own peers. Except for a few stalwarts like Dr Elizabeth Blackwell, women did not break through this barrier. Reformed nursing, in spite of the high regard in which it was held, was seen more as a vocation than as a profession, and Miss Nightingale herself was insistent that her trainees should put 'vocation' first and was fearful of nursing being seen on a narrow commercial basis. However, words change their meaning, and both Miss Nightingale and her contemporaries seem to use 'vocation' and 'profession' in different senses at different times. But in the nineteenth century sense nursing did not qualify as a profession, nurses were *not* independent practitioners and indeed, the insistence on obedience was anti-ethical to independence and self sufficiency.

During the twentieth century the influence of new ideologies, the growth of technology, and the impact of two world wars have led not only to a more egalitarian society, but to new ideas about the value of different occupations, although, curiously enough the differentials between the older professions and other groups remain perversely the same.

By a strange paradox there has been an increasing demand for entry to the professions to be enlarged. Bernard Shaw's eminent barrister, Mr Bohum, in 'You Never Can Tell'[2] was the son of the hotel waiter; this is how the Fabian socialists saw the achievement of equality of opportunity—not by democracy but by better opportunities for education. But the limitations of the educational system and the increase in the level of knowledge demanded for entrants into the professions, of which the medical profession is a prime example, has meant that entry has remained limited. On the other hand, the rising cost of technology and the pressure for a fairer distribution of services such as education and health, has led to more and more of these services being supplied by public administration, and ipso facto, professional men and women are 'employed' like other workers. In these circumstances professional workers may experience a conflict between the demands of their employers and the aims of their profession. For example, employers often want information whereas the professional code requires confidentiality. Finally, the situation has been further confused by continual changes in the legislation concerning industrial relations and, from this point of view, a lack of clear distinction between trade unions and professional organisations.

The Characteristics of a Profession

In her book *The Professional Ethic*[3] Norah Mackenzie, using the writings of R. M. McIver, C. M. Page, Sir Harold Himsworth, Professor Whithead and Plato, deduced 15 separate characteristics of a profession. Setting aside Plato's eternal verity that a profession is the "pursuit of excellence" and that "the physician studies only the patient's interest, not his own",[4] these are characteristics which are for the most part subsumed in the two main points within Sir Harold Himsworth's now classic lecture to the Medical Research Council.

Sir Harold works from the premiss that for a profession to exist there has to be a particular need in society, and a recognition by society that the body of men and women undertaking to meet this need must be given special recognition. In other words a tacit social contract is implied: "obligation on the part of society to afford the professional man such status, authority and privilege as shall be required for him to discharge his obligations. Only in so far and for so long as this implied contract is observed will the profession in question survive".[5] For example, for a doctor to be able to meet the health needs of the community, society must agree that he can carry dangerous drugs and make incisions into the human body, which, for persons not so privileged, would be an offence against the law. Similiarly, lawyers must be allowed access to information and not be forced to disclose it by law, because only in this way, and with this privilege, can they gain the confidence of their clients. Generally speaking, the greater the privilege to be above the law, the greater the responsibility and the greater the reward.

If professions have an implied contract with society which gives them 'status, authority and privilege' then society wants certain assurances in return. If doctors can order their patients dangerous drugs or lawyers be responsible for clients' money, the public want to know that the training and skill of these privileged people is of the best. But skill is not enough, there must also be a code of ethics which indicates how clients and patients should be served and the attitudes that should be accepted. Nurses, for example, accept that health is a basic human right regardless of colour, race or creed, and solicitors than justice is a fundamental in an ordered society. Clearly no one should enter a profession without subscribing to its fundamental tenets.

The first hallmark of a profession then is that it embodies *competence and skill that is more than ordinary*. On this point Sir Harold is worth quoting in full. In answer to the question "What is it that society needs from a profession?" he says:

"Firstly, it requires special competence — the technical skill to meet, to an ever increasing extent, the needs which called the profession into existence. In law that requires competence in applying and interpreting the rules of conduct in a particular society; in teaching it requires acquisition of knowledge and skill to impart it; in medicine it implies competence to preserve health and treat illness. Unless society has the requisite degree of confidence in the technical competence of its professions they are helpless. And what is that degree? In the professions the standard of competence required to elicit public confidence is never ordinary. The needs to be met are too vital to survive the suspicion that the best has not been available. It is this that makes the continual prosecution of research an essential factor in maintaining public confidence in our professions. It is this that makes the continual striving after excellence, rather than mere competence, the criterion of professional endeavour."

But Sir Harold goes on to point out that praiseworthy though all this is, it might apply to any skilled occupation — designing computers, for example. But it is not skill, nor yet esoteric language, that distinguishes the professions in the eyes of the man in the street. Mere skill does not command affection. There is therefore another characteristic, more difficult to define, but it relates not to what the practitioner knows but to the kind of person he or she is.

The reason for this is not far to seek. To quote Bernard Shaw again "All professions are a conspiracy against the laity"[6] and as medicine, and its allied professions, become more advanced and its language more unintelligible even to the educated public, how *can* people know that their own personal good is not being sacrificed to the general good, or to the advancement of the profession? With every further specialisation the ordinary man is more vulnerable. How can he be sure that he is a suitable subject for a transplant, and is this best for him? The answer is he can only trust. But what inspires trust?

Sir Harold goes on:

"Such trust can only come from voluntary acts which augment confidence . . . there is no more potent stimulus to this than that of a man — or a body of men, voluntarily submitting themselves to a standard of social morality more exacting than that required by the community in general. Such voluntary subordination is the hallmark of those vocations that are commonly distinguished as professions. It is this that accounts for the special respect in which they are held and the privileges which they are accorded."

Professional men and women, therefore, must act always so as to increase trust, and this is why professions have their own disciplinary bodies which have the power to remove the names of practitioners who destroy trust, either because they are professionally incompetent, or, more controversially, because personal behaviour makes them unworthy of that trust.

Professional Discipline

People have argued that Professional Disciplinary Committees are an anachronism in the modern world. Professional competence has been tested by qualification, and registration is given only to safe practitioners. Now that so many professional people are employed by an authority, if they become unsafe or incompetent they can be fairly dismissed (see Chapter 7). This argument is not valid because in fact not all professionals are employed by an authority and, secondly, if an employee is dismissed for incompetence the public are not protected because the dismissed person can apply for, and probably get, another job. References are too often guarded, and management are not always clear about their legal position and fear a come-back, and the employing authority is not always as careful as it should be about checking references.

However, it is not the first hallmark of the profession which so often exercises the Professional Disciplinary Committees but the second, that there has been professional misconduct which is in some way morally blameworthy but which may, or may not be, legally wrong.

"An action taken by a doctor may be neither contrary to the law nor to the regulations governing the National Health Service and yet may be considered unethical by his colleagues as to constitute grounds for a formal complaint to the Association".[7]

The same principle is valid for nurses who are reported to the Disciplinary Committee of what was the General Nursing Council and is now the United Kingdom Central Council for Nursing, Midwifery and Health Visiting (UKCC). While a number of cases involve offences that are legally wrong—such as the stealing of drugs or the taking of controlled drugs that have not been prescribed, or shoplifting—others, like relationships with patients, may not be legally wrong but, nevertheless, might be such as to render the practitioner, in the eyes of his peers, to be a 'not fit and proper person'. Much depends on the nature of the offence and whether or not it destroys trust. The defitting conduct that most often causes solicitors to be struck off the Roll is the using of client's money for their own purposes; for doctors and nurses it is often because of the misuse of drugs: in this case there has been not only an offence at law but an abuse of the profession's special privilege. However, the abuse of a professional relationship with a patient is often not a legal offence but it is an abuse of privilege and trust and as such could bring the profession in question into disrepute.

So serious is the removal of a name from a Register or Roll that rights of appeal are laid down by Acts of Parliament and the rules made under them. *The Nurses Act 1970* gives the right of appeal to the High Court, while doctors, dentists and the professions supplementary to medicine, can appeal to the judicial committee of the Privy Council. Disciplinary Committees must observe the natural rules of justice, but although they can compel attendance of witnesses they are not bound by the rules of evidence and they are usually more relaxed than a law court. Although an appeal from a professional body is technically possible, in practice such judgements are seldom set aside.

Over the years the nature of the offences reported to the Council has changed; this is partly due to the changing mores of society, for example, neither adultery nor giving birth to an illegitimate child attracts the opprobrium it once did. In some cases, however, it is because the law itself has changed, good examples being the law on abortion and on homosexual offences. Nevertheless, the number of cases appearing before the Council is increasing; this is, of course, partly due to an absolute increase in the number of nurses, and possibly because the work of the Council in this respect is better known. However, this increase is worth pondering and it is worth listing the reasons the Assistant Registrar sees as the reasons for the relative increase in the cases appearing before the Council.[8] Firstly, some nurses, and often the most willing, are allowed by their superiors—and sometimes encouraged by them, to accept an impossible workload. All too often nurse managers fail to protest when financial cuts or staff shortages mean that it is no longer possible to carry out safe nursing practice. The second reason refers to the extended role of the nurse and the fact that this is sometimes accepted without proper precautions (see Chapter 4).

Apart from these reasons it is clear that many nurses come before the Court because they are sick and preventive measures have not been taken in time. Although since 1972 there has been a welfare service attached to the Council for cases referred to them, this is all too often a closing of the stable door after the horse has gone. Prevention needs to start earlier; the basic nursing education should give more time to making students aware of what it means to be a member of a profession and to the fact that they are both morally and legally accountable for their professional acts. This understanding of accountability is now more urgent because with the increasing use of the nursing process where nurses assess, plan, implement and evaluate nursing care, they are independent practitioners, and, if they expect to be regarded as such, they must accept the responsibility that is the concomitant of that expectation.

Apart from the need to give students this understanding early in their training, nurse managers and educators have a duty to create a dynamic work setting where all practitioners are given the opportunity of furthering their professional knowledge and seeing their education as a continual process. However, there is another failure. Many of the cases that come before the Council, and often those people who seek help from their professional organisations, illustrate the need for a better occupational health service in the National Health Service. All too often the cobbler's children are the worst shod and there is a need for more awareness of the professional and domestic pressures to which many nurses are subjected to in their daily lives.

Finally, while it is the first duty of every nurse to be, and to remain, a safe practitioner, and be a fit and proper person, accidents and complications happen and all nurses should have access to independent advice and counselling. Apart from representing members who face disciplinary action from their employers or professional body, most organisations for employees offer a welfare service. The Royal College of Nursing has CHAT (Counselling Help and Advice Together) which is a personal advisory service for nurses and gives confidential help on a wide range of questions. It is important that not only is help available but that it is known to be available. Nurses have attempted suicide in despair, not because the help they needed was not there, but because they did not know it was there.

Is Nursing a Profession?

Nursing has acknowledged the two main hallmarks of a profession. After 1919 it required the practitioner to give evidence of a certain standard before 'registration', after which the title nurse was legally (although not actually) reserved for those so registered. The public were therefore assured of a certain standard of skill *at the time of registration.* In 1925 the General Nursing Council set up a Disciplinary Committee empowered to remove the name of any nurse who was deemed not 'a fit and proper person' and, in the intervening years, has done so.

Although nursing apparently meets the two main hallmarks of a profession, areas of doubt remain. When the Nightingale Fund Council argued against the concept of registration before the Privy Council in 1891, it made the point that it was merely a test of a nurse's knowledge on a particular day and it would offer no safeguard for the public, or the new profession of nursing unless there could be continual assessment. This argument is still valid.

Apart from this, many people have argued that nursing has no special competence but consists merely of eclectic borrowings from other disciplines; but this is true of all the newer professions — social science amongst them; basically they are all derived from theology, philosophy and medicine. It is not the hybrid nature of nursing that is open to question but the fact that, until recently, nursing has failed to build up a unique body of knowledge and to base its practices on scientific research. What is interesting, and historically paradoxical, is that at the beginning of the twentieth century when nursing was making much fuss about being a profession and being 'registered', it was becoming, in the large general hospitals at least, the handmaiden of medicine in a way that it had never been before.

This argument is losing its force because demographic change is now such that many people who now need nursing care suffer from defects or disabilities for which medicine can do little, and which could not have been reasonably prevented and now cannot be cured. What is left is care. Experimental Nursing Homes have recently been opened in the charge of nurses who prescribe care and call the general practitioner as appropriate. This nursing approach has been urged not only in this country but in the United States where, of course, cost effectiveness is even more important to the individual patient.[9]

Because of these changes in the health needs of the population, and because of the fact that nurses are now prescribing care, there is a considerable body of research being built into nursing practice, although until nurse training is on a more heuristic basis these findings are not likely to be widely used. There has, for example, been much research into the prevention of pressure sores, but until recently few nursing histories seemed to include the Norton Scale. Notwithstanding these failings, there is an increasing commitment in both basic and post basic education — supported by space in nursing journals, to study nursing problems and models rather than the sociological and medical models so favoured in the past. In this respect the Nursing Process can be said to be post hoc ergo propter hoc, and a response to changed health needs. When this system is better understood it should lead to the substitution of the scientific method for folklore, the prescribing of care on a

personal basis, and should go some way to meeting that require-
ment of a profession that it builds up knowledge by "the
continual prosecution of research".

Another pointer to the growing professionalism of nursing is
that it is developing a number of nursing specialisms as opposed
to specialised nursing as a response to various medical specialities.
Good examples of 'nursing' specialisms are terminal care
nursing, stoma therapy and infection control—these studies are
aimed at producing better ways of prescribing nursing care over
a wide range of different medical specialities.

Accountability in Nursing

Apart from the failure to be research minded and to build up a
body of nursing knowledge based on research, nurses have been
criticised, and rightly so, for not seeing themselves as professional
practitioners and responsible for their own professional acts; the
nurse's confusion has been confounded by the different
perceptions of the nurse's role by doctors on the one hand and
lay administrators on the other.[10] Only now, when the
techniques performed by nurses (often taken over from the
doctor) are potentially more dangerous, are doctors dissuaded
from saying that *they* are responsible for techniques performed
by nurses.

This confusion has its roots in history. When Miss Nightingale
started her 'reformed nurse training' the emphasis was on
practical training, and although there were some lectures from
doctors, the important instruction was supposed to be on the
wards. In order to achieve this, the Nightingale Fund paid part
of the salaries of the 'training sisters' and the matron, and they
insisted that the control of the nurses should be in the hands of
'a trained female superintendent'. This was not instituting a
'hierarchy' as some people have suggested but of wresting the
power of hiring and firing from the doctors and the chaplains.
Nurses were now accountable to another nurse. However, within
a decade or so the germ theory of infection was validated and
medicine became more scientific. Where better could doctors
find assistants than from the ranks of the highly disciplined and
trustworthy reformed nurses, to whom they now gave lectures in

chemistry and physics? Increasingly nurses were giving injections and doing the treatment once done by doctors. Above all they were becoming the doctor's eyes and, with the aid of tools like thermometers, urine testing agents and the sphygmomanometer, they took over many of the measuring and analysing tasks. In general hospitals nurses now worked more and more with doctors to whom they were rightly responsible for treatment, but they were accountable to, and controlled by, the nursing superintendent. It is small wonder that many nurses were ambivalent about their responsibility and accountability.

Although there were occasional conflicts between the matron and the doctors about what nurses should do, before the coming of the National Health Service this caused little real trouble. Few people ever sued hospitals and the legal aspect was less important. Now the situation has changed and the role of the nurse has extended and is likely to extend further, the health service is paid for by taxation and is likely to be sued like any other public enterprise. Professor T. McKeown has suggested that "the traditional roles of doctors and nurses in primary care may now be inappropriate" and "that the nurse is capable of giving a service which in some countries the physician seems unable or unwilling to provide."[11] If Professor McKeown is right, ambiguity about responsibility and accountability would be disastrous.

The Social Contract and the Right to Protest

If a profession is a group with a social contract with society then the contract implies that there are two sides to the bargain. There may be times when the profession feels that society has not kept its part of the contract; this does not only apply to monetary reward but to the 'authority and status' mentioned earlier. There may come a point where reward for service is so low that the profession is unable to recruit, or to retain, suitable candidates. In the past this has actually been true for nursing, although it is less likely to prove a good argument in a time of high unemployment. On the other hand, there may be cases where the rewards are reasonable but that the conditions are so poor that the best endeavours are frustrated. Examples could be long hours for junior doctors and the inadequate coverage on night duty for nurses. In these circumstances the profession has a duty to protest in the interest of the greater good.

The problem now arises, how to protest and to whom? Obviously, extreme methods should not be contemplated until all constitutional and democratic channels have been explored. A number of questions have to be asked. Firstly, what is the real consensus of the group as a whole? Often this is not easily known. Secondly, how urgent is the situation in terms of falling standards and a failure to recruit, and is this 'fall' based on factual evidence? Thirdly, to what extent has the group fallen behind comparable groups in economic rewards and, of course, what is comparable? Fourthly, what are the exceptional responsibilities borne by the group—are they 'a special case' and what is the standard of entry required of candidates to meet these responsibilities. Fifthly, is the claim 'reasonable' and is there any hope of getting the necessary manpower or finance? For example, it is no use demanding ever more nurses in a time of full employment when the only way they can be obtained is by depleting other services. Nor is it any use taking money from other public servcies, for the social services are so interlocked that the failure of one immediately throws a strain on the others. Low pensions mean more cases admitted with hypothermia. It is no use pushing back the hand of death with new, expensive technology if there is no money for some quality of life for those to whom the added years have been given. Nor, indeed, would the health services be helped if they took money from education, since health is now largely a matter of intelligent self help and an understanding of the issues involved.

Finally, professional and economic considerations should not be mixed with political issues; if they are both causes may be damaged, this is particularly true of secondary picketing as the health service strikes in the 'winter of discontent' illustrated; the public on the whole take unkindly to being held to ransom on political issues. However, it is possible to conceive of circumstances where strikes and withdrawal of labour for political reasons are justifiable, for example where liberty is being curtailed in a totalitarian state, but in a democracy the strike weapon should not be used instead of the ballot box and the hustings.

It is, however, a commonplace that in a time of rapid inflation the public services lose out at the expense of the private sector. Tracing the economic fortunes of the nursing profession over the past forty years it is not without significance that nurses tend to gain during a period of an 'incomes policy' and to lose in a rapid free for all.[12]

Recently, partly because enterprises like the National Health Service have looked to industry for management help and industrial relations 'know-how', there has been an increasing tendency to think that all the methods used in the industrial situation can be applied to a public service, and that grievances will be settled if labour is withdrawn. Apart from the ethical considerations, withdrawing labour from the mines or the electricity generating stations has a very different practical implication, the most important being that a stoppage of work means a loss of profit and negotiations take place under economic pressure on the management. In extreme cases, as with electricity, the nation could be held to ransom. Not so with the social and health services. Withdrawing services from the sick does not exert economic pressure; indeed if hospitals were closed the government would save money. Generally speaking, withdrawal of labour from a public service—even the Post Office—has no industrial power; it does not cause a run on the pound nor yet effect the Stock Market. It can, of course, have a nuisance value but in the Health Services this is likely to be comparatively ineffective on two counts. Firstly, unless the disaffected are prepared to put pickets on the emergency services and intensive care, there would probably be enough volunteers to carry on without more disruption than the public could bear. Moreover, who is to say what is urgent? How do laboratory workers know which tests are urgent until they have been analysed? How do you know which cases in casualty are 'urgent' until they have been examined? Secondly, as a method of protest for withdrawal of labour to be effective, it must be pushed to the point where the sick and the vulnerable actually suffer harm and lives are put in danger. Apart from the morality of such a course it would be self-defeating, public trust would be lost, and it is the public who pay. "Harming the weak and sick is not the best way of pursuading society to pay higher taxes."

In the seven years since those words were written in the first edition they have been forcibly illustrated. In 1978 the social workers in Southwark went on strike, a strike that was largely ignored by the press, in fact there was some questioning by the press about the value of social workers—did we need them? Then in an article 'We Three Kings of Misery Are'[13] *The Guardian* drew attention to a reversal of the usual ritual about the attitude of unions to a strike. Generally they were at pains to *deny* stories about 'little old ladies freezing to death or dangerously sick patients failing to reach hospital' and they usually made a real effort to protect the most vulnerable. But now a "caring profession" actually issued a document proclaiming that 'the conditions of children in care were at explosion point and that the elderly sick were in danger, and those who think the social services are unnecessary should think again".

This was hardly the way to win friends, but the social workers were in a Catch 22 situation which the professions enter at their peril. Although the situation only applied to a few workers who, presumably, had a genuine grievance, the outcome of ill will and bad press was out of all proportion to the harm that may have been done. When cuts have to be made the strike is remembered. There is always the danger that we will not be missed as much as we think.

Finally, there is the legal consideration. Technically speaking, withdrawal of labour constitutes a breach of contract and can be a reason for dismissal. Although the *Employment Protection Act 1975* (see Chapter 7) lays down safeguards concerning such action in the pursuance of a bona fide trade union activity, much would depend on the particular circumstances, and an 'unofficial' walk-out where patients were left without cover might well be tested as a case for fair dismissal.

Furthermore, if patients suffered avoidable harm as the result of the withdrawal of labour by nurses, the well-advised patient, or his relatives, might sue the hospital and the onus of blame could be put on the person, or persons, who were absent without leave. Whatever the outcome, the publicity would be undesirable and public trust would be lost.

On ethical, legal and practical grounds therefore, the strike weapon is unsuitable as a means of protest by professional practitioners and they have to use other ways of making their point.

In the first place there is no substitute for a case well presented and well argued, backed by factual evidence. Ultimately decisions are made at the conference table and not in the street, but since it is the public who will pay for the services and the salaries they must be kept informed, and, generally speaking, if the facts are properly presented the public know a hawk from a handsaw. This may mean mounting a public relations exercise, which seems time-consuming compared with industrial action, but it has paid off in the past, and it can pay dividends and if it does the gains are great because whatever they are they are made without loss of public respect. In the last resort the public gets the health, or any other service, for which it is prepared to pay. Society having willed the ends must also will the means.

References

1 TUC Health Services Committee (1981) *Improving Industrial Relations in the National Health Service*. London TUC Publications, p.119

2 Shaw G. B. (1896) *You Never Can Tell, Act IV*. London: Odhams Press

3 Mackenzie N. (1971) *The Professional Ethic*. London: English Universities Press

4 Plato *The Republic*. Intro. 1976 ed., trans Desmond Lee. Harmondsworth; Penguin Books

5 Himsworth H. (1953) Change and permanence in education for medicine. *Lancet* **ii**, 789

6 Shaw G. B. (1905) *The Doctor's Dilemma*. London: Odhams Press

7 British Medical Association (1963) *Handbook*. Quoted Whincup N. H. (1982) *Legal Aspects of Medical and Nursing Services*. Beckenham: Ravenswood Press

8 Pyne R. (1971) *Professional Discipline in Nursing*. Oxford: Blackwell Scientific Publications

9 Copp L. A. Ed. (1981) *Care of the Aging*. Edinburgh: Churchill Livingstone, Ch. 6

10   Anderson E. R. (1973) *The Role of the Nurse.* RCN Research
     Series 2, No.1 London: Royal College of Nursing
11   McKeown T. (1976) *The Role of Medicine.* London:
     Nuffield Provincial Hospitals Trust, p.121
12   Baly M. E. (1980) *Nursing and Social Change.* London:
     Heinemann Medical Books, pp.371–377
13   The Guardian (1978) *Leader*, 23 December

Chapter 2

Social Change and
New Health Needs

If there is a tacit contract between the professions and society, it
follows that the professions, and their responsibilities, must
change as the needs of society change. Before examining the
specific professional responsibilities and the ethical and legal
problems that confront health workers it is worth looking at how,
and why, the needs of society have changed. Without this understanding it is impossible for workers to make a sensitive response.

Apart from the responsibility for continual research, the
result of which may change the whole direction of a profession,
as did the discovery of the germ theory of infection, it is a
hallmark of a profession that it accepts the responsibility itself
for adapting its educational programme to meet new needs. In a
time of rapid social change this is by no means easy. This
chapter seeks to give a brief outline of how and why the health
needs of the community have changed during this century, and
how the services have adapted — or failed to adapt — to meet
those needs, and to question whether the health professions, and
particularly nursing, have, and are, adapting quickly enough.
Those who perhaps feel that understanding social change is not
part of the responsibility of the profession should study the
content of the syllabus for basic nurse training, or indeed any
nursing syllabus during the first two decades of the National
Health Service and ask if they really prepared nurses to meet the
new health needs.

Social Change

Many factors interact in producing social change; for example,
demographic change both produces social change and is itself

19

caused by social and economic changes, but as the population profile is paramount in dictating the health needs of the community it is convenient to start at this point in the circle.

Demographic Transition

After centuries of an almost stable population with very slow growth, since the middle of the eighteenth century there have been two startling disruptions. Firstly, there was the unprecedented population increase starting round about 1750 (see Figure 1) which was an important factor in both the industrial and the French revolutions—an example of the circularity of cause and effect in social change. The reasons for this increase are still partly obscure, but an important factor was the improved food supply brought about by the agrarian revolution and the increased trade with the colonies.[1] This was assisted by a series of good harvests and the fact that there were no major epidemics, and finally, there was a marginal improvement in urban hygiene. The population rose from 6 million in 1700 to 18 million in 1850. It was this threefold increase that made governments fear that the gloomy prognostications of Thomas Malthus were coming true. It is worth recalling this because as legislators coped with the new needs of the increased urban population in a piecemeal and unplanned manner they laid the foundations of our present health services —a foundation that still effects resource allocation and attitudes.

The population increase both fed the industrial revolution and provided its market. There was a cyclic situation with population pressure, technological invention and the resources available, pursuing one another in ever widening circles, a situation now to be found in parts of the third world. But growth carried its own contradictions in terms of 'booms' then saturated markets and cyclic unemployment, and it is doubtful if the standard of living was markedly improved for many workers until the second half of the nineteenth century.[2] By the middle of that century rapid urbanisation in the industrial areas had led to house building without proper sanitation and overcrowding which was the predisposing factor in the water-borne epidemics of the mid century, the most devastating of which was cholera.

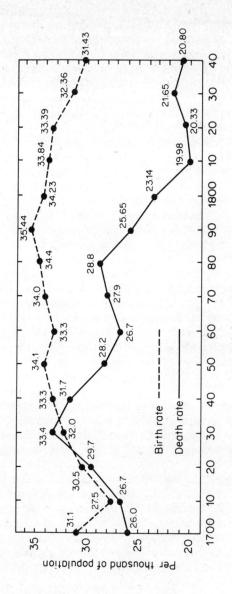

Figure 1. Rates of birth and death in the 18th century. (Reproduced, with acknowledgement from *Population Problems of the Age of Malthus*. G. Talbot Griffith, Cambridge University Press, 1962)

It was these epidemics which caused the hiccough in the death rate shown in Figure 1. The response was the sanitary campaigns of men like Edwin Chadwick, John Simon and the early medical officers of health which led eventually to supplies of clean water, the removal of effluvia by more hygienic methods and, that greatest of all blessings to health, the water closet. By the end of the century epidemics of water-borne diseases had been eliminated but other health problems had taken their place; sanitation had not brought the millenium.

In the mid 1880s faith in the continual progress of industry was shattered by the great depression largely caused by competition from the newly industrialised countries; the English industrial revolution was running out of steam. This caused periods of high unemployment and although wages were still improving there was increasing abject poverty. This is the background of Booth's Survey of 1899–1902 *Life and Labour of People in London* and Seebohm Rowntree's survey of York in 1908 *Poverty: A Study of Town Life*. Both surveys suggested that one third of the population was living below the "poverty line", a new concept of Charles Booth's own devising. This poverty was the main reason why the infant mortality rate stood at around 156 per 1000 live births — an example of the effect of the economy on the demographic picture.

With the validation of the germ theory of infection, much of this ill health and death — and particularly child death — was seen as preventable and steps could be taken to meet the challenge. A landslide victory in 1905 gave the Liberal government a chance to introduce a mass of social and health legislation which is important because it is the matrix of the present health and welfare services. This is a further example of our health services heritage designed to meet the needs of a different era.

Legislation included the notification of infectious diseases, the notification of births — with the subsequent development of health visiting emphasising the care of mothers and babies; in 1906 school meals were introduced, and the following year school medical inspections. Already in 1902, the *Midwives Act* had ensured that midwives received a training and were 'certificated'. 1908 saw the first *Old Age Pension Act* and 1911

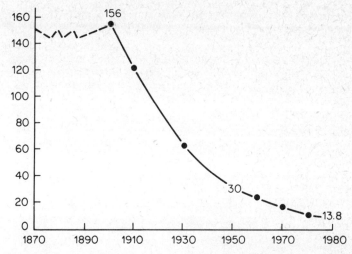

Figure 2. Infant mortality rates in England and Wales. (Reproduced in amended form from Baly M. E. 1980 *Nursing and Social Change*. London: William Heinemann Medical Books)

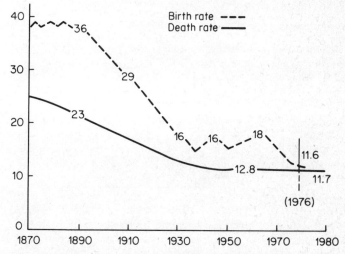

Figure 3. Birth and death rates per 1000 population in England and Wales. (Reproduced in amended form from Baly M. E. 1980 *Nursing and Social Change*. London: William Heinemann Medical Books)

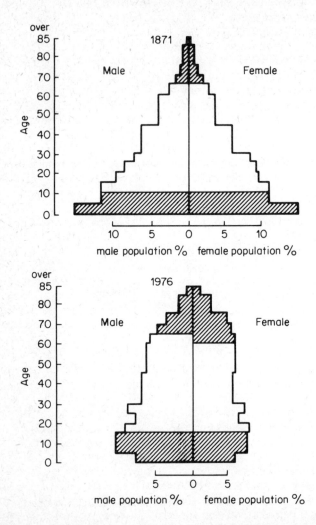

Figure 4. Population profiles, 1871 and 1976; shaded areas indicate non-workers. (Reproduced from Baly M. E. 1980 *Nursing and Social Change*. London: William Heinemann Medical Books)

The National Insurance Act which was in fact the foundation stone of the Beveridge Report.

There are many interrelating reasons for the next dramatic demographic change (Figures 2 and 3) and, although improvement in health was due mainly to causes outside medical care, some of the reasons are not unconnected with the legislation outlined in the previous paragraph. Firstly, the high birth rate fell because large families were no longer an economic asset. The Factory Acts of 1844, 1847, 1867 and 1878 had decreased the value of child labour, and compulsory education after the *Education Act* 1902 meant that children were now an economic liability. However, perhaps the most powerful reason for the fall in the birth rate derived from the fact that better midwifery, health and social services had lowered the infant mortality rate and the need for replacement was less. Bound with this was the movement for the emancipation of women and the work of pioneers like Marie Stopes in family planning which helped the voluntary limitation of family size. This interlocking of many reasons, including the social unrest before the First World War, brought about the most dramatic change in the population profile since the plague epidemics of the fourteenth century. Within a space of 40 years the birth and death rates were halved, with profound effects not only on the demographic pattern, but on the demands for health services.

In 1901 there were one and a half million people past retirement age: today there are nine million, representing about 16 per cent of the population. Not only are there more people in retirement, but there is an increase in the proportion of the population over 75 and over 85 years old, and these groups make the heaviest demands on the health and social services.[3] A number of other consequences have flowed from the fall in the infant death rate. When there is a high infant death rate more boy babies die than girls; once the death rate is cut there is a tendency for the ratio to be equal. There are then fewer surplus girls and marriage tends to take place earlier with the child-bearing period completed sooner. This being so, more wives are able to work outside the home and for longer periods which has important consequences for the supply of recruits to nursing and, conversely, on the demand for nursing services.

The development of nursing to meet new needs since the middle of the nineteenth century has been pragmatic. Early reformed nursing concentrated mainly on developing a nursing service to give care to the poor sick in hospitals and infirmaries and in the homes of the poor 'on the district'. However, it should be remembered that without the benefits of registration or professional organisation, nursing did develop specialities to meet new needs. It is arguable whether in the post-Second-World-War period, nursing, with all its organisational advantages, developed a geriatric nursing service as quickly as the nurses at the beginning of the century developed a 'Fever Nursing' service or a 'Children's Nursing' service.

Men and Women at Work

Almost as important as the changed demographic structure is the changed pattern of work. How and where people work affects their health and the kind of demand they make on the health services. Once, most of the population were engaged in some form of farming or fishing, now the proportion is less than 3 per cent. In the late nineteenth century the highest proportion were employed in manufacturing; now it is only 30 per cent. The rest are employed mainly in the service industries, with between 6 and 7 per cent in public administration and the health services accounting for 1·2 million out of a total work force of 24 million (5 per cent).[4] These occupations may be cleaner than grinding or mining but they carry their own problems as is shown by the fact that the life expectation for men at the age of 45 years has not improved in the last 80 years.[4] However, it is important to remember that a tenth of all working days lost is due to illness from a prescribed disease.

Apart from the tensions associated with modern travel and the communications system, perhaps the greatest problem now is not so much work but, as micro-electronics revolutionise more and more industries, the fear of being without work. In the nineteenth century the stockingers, whose skills were displaced by new machines, took hammers and smashed the machines; it did not halt the revolution but it was a symbolic gesture of how people feel when deprived of work and of using their particular skill. Today, displaced workers do not use hammers but the frustration is still there, and for a society geared to the work ethic, unemployment can have consequences for mental and physical health. Research is currently being undertaken but earlier studies have already shown that families are particularly vulnerable when unemployment is combined with such things as personality difficulties and large families.

Housing Patterns

These are often related to other factors such as demographic change, although it is significant that neither the private nor the public sector has done much to meet the housing needs of older citizens, many of whom live alone. Housing is, of course, greatly influenced by where people work. For example, the great increase in the number of people working in offices means that more people can live in the suburbs. In the last 60 years the housing stock has altered radically with the peak alterations following the two world wars. After the First World War, new housing was largely ribbon development, the results of which are still with us. After the Second World War there was a determination to avoid the unplanned sprawl of the inter-war years and a new policy for housing was developed based on slum clearance and a new social cohesion. Whole areas were cleared in the cities and the occupants rehoused in tower blocks which were linked to road networks. Originally it was intended that the areas between the blocks should have trees, gardens and a variety of amenities thus creating a new 'neighbourhood', meeting, as it were, on the village green. Unfortunately, the end results seldom looked like the architect's drawings. Designed to meet the needs of the nuclear family it was thought that each block would provide a sense of community and that central maintenance would ensure a standard of hygiene. What was not foreseen was that a panoramic view over the docklands did not compensate for the claustrophobia, the invitation to vandalism and the appalling maintenance costs. The new 'prisons in the sky' have been unpopular with old people who fear being trapped when the lift breaks down, and mothers with young babies who feel utterly isolated. Statistics show that dwellers in tower blocks have more health and social problems than people in other types of housing, and some have an unduly high record of visits from the probation officer.

Meanwhile, convenient bomb damage gave developers a chance to turn city centres over to profitable office blocks, hotels and shops while the displaced population—with not enough points for a place in a tower block—move to the next concentric circle, the twilight zone of the inner city. Because of the decay of these areas they are often scheduled for redevelopment or destruction, and 'planning blight' means that they are badly provided for by the services they most need. Local authorities do not build health centres when they contemplate using a bulldozer.

Housing, like work, has a bearing on health, and it is the health worker's continuing professional responsibility to be aware of housing legislation and, in the case of the health workers in the community, to be their patients' advocates when housing conditions affect their health. *Home from Hospital*[5] showed all too well that hospital workers were often woefully unaware of the conditions to which they were returning vulnerable patients.

But not all patients live in cities: many live on Council estates of varying degrees of modernity, which the practised eye of a health visitor can usually date within a few years, and in spite of blandishments there seems little likelihood of a great deal of this stock being transferred to private ownership. However, almost two-thirds of the population live in private housing, mostly owner occupied, and sometimes heavily mortgaged. But even in the leafy suburbs houses are seldom designed for more than the nuclear family, and, with fitted labour-saving devices they are a positive incentive to wives of all classes to work, gainfully or otherwise, outside the home. These two factors make it difficult for children to take in elderly parents even if both parties wished it—which they usually do not. Moreover, sheer longevity makes it less feasible than formerly. Widowed, or single daughters aged 70 years can be found coping with mothers in their 90s. Nor should it be forgotten that middle class housing is increasingly sheltering ageing widows or single women who often become lonely and socially withdrawn and are less likely to be known intimately by their neighbours than people in villages or old working class areas. Such people, when failing, need the services of the health visitor or the district nurse as much as the poor sick of former years, and they need as much sensitive consideration when they are discharged from hospital. Society has abolished the servant class and money cannot buy the domestic help so often needed.

There is another housing pattern that must loom large in the community health worker's case load, that of the retirement areas. Now that both men and women have pensions they plan their retirement, which may be nearly as long as their working life. Often they move to retirement areas, perhaps bungalows by the sea, surrounded by other retired couples. Usually they are fitter than previous generations and for a time they are the valuable allies of the community health workers. They are the drivers of 'meals on wheels', the workers for fund raising without which the health services would not only be materially poorer but poorer in spirit. Unfortunately, the discrepancy between the male and female life expectancy rates means that such areas have a prepondenance of widows, who, when health fails, or they become forgetful or disorientated, are now removed from their families; the grass grows higher and the trees encroach on the once sunny bungalow sitting room. It is not that the children do not care, but with small families there are fewer to bear the burden and people must go where the work is, so when the only son is working on an oil rig in the North Sea and the two grandchildren are at universities in the north of England they are not much help when grandmother has a stroke in Bognor.

Economic Changes

Some recent economic changes are related to changing work patterns and demographic change. One obvious fact is that 42 per cent of all married women now work outside the home and many family budgets are geared to two incomes, and the things that the family now buys in the supermarket were once made in the home. In spite of England's poor economic performance as compared with competitor countries, most people have experienced a rise in the standard of living. However, it must be remembered that what we regard as an adequate standard must be measured by what society today regards as a 'norm', not what was the 'norm' for the Booth survey.[6] But in spite of the real benefits of the Welfare State groups in society have remained unequal in their opportunities, and since the oil crisis of 1973, and more recently with the dramatic rise in unemployment, real poverty is again often an underlying factor in ill health. The question of poverty, its causes and effects, have been extensively debated by such researchers as Titmuss, Townsend, Abel Smith, Rein and Berthoud all of whom call into question the traditional attitudes to poverty.

What must concern the health worker is the fact that universal health and educational services have not brought equal opportunities to children of low income families. Children from homes where there are books and opportunities for going to places of interest and the live theatre do better at school than children from homes without these advantages. As Berthoud shows,[7] the children are more likely to go to universities, to get better jobs, suffer less ill health and less hardship when they are ill than low income families. Status often effects where people live, and children are more likely to do well if they are brought up in Bromley than in Brixton. Of particular interest to the health visitor are the findings of the Black Report of 1980, *Inequalities of Health*, which showed that although people in Social Class V consulted their general practitioners more often, and were heavier users of hospital beds, they made less use of the preventive services. This difference in usage is also true of the use of the dental services, the family planning services, and markedly true of the school health services, where it was found that they were used more by parents in the higher socio-economic groups who were anxious for their children to be healthy and who could talk freely with the doctor and the nurse. Now, the neglected Black report is vindicated by later research, *Despite the Welfare State*,[8] which shows that in the family life of the poor the cycle of deprivation continues to operate. Inequalities are seen across a wide spectrum such as the use of public libraries, adult evening education. Keep Fit classes — used mostly by the fit — and the take up of opportunities offered by the Open University. The failure to serve those in most need has caused much heart searching among the social scientists and in some cases there have been suggestions for positive inverse discrimination as in the recommendations of the Plowden Report and, more recently, the Scarman Report. However, when it comes to the failure of the use of the preventive services by the most vulnerable groups in society, the health visitors of yesteryear need to ask themselves some very searching questions about their professional responsibility. Were they too well prepared for grateful clients, and insufficiently for the alienated section of society for whom the health services, and the professional worker who comes to see them, are a middle class concept and to be avoided? If we have failed we must ask ourselves why, and press for a change in the preparation of health workers so that these pitfalls, inasfar as they can be avoided, are avoided.

Lifestyles

Changed work patterns and economic circumstances, more consumer choice, the effect of television, universal education to 16 years and more adolescents going on to higher education have had a profound effect on the way people live, what they want from their lives and what they expect from the public services. It is only necessary to look at the role model offered to brides-to-be in the popular magazines of the 1930s and compare it with the media appeal to the same age groups today to realise the profound change.

The mass media has effected the way people use their leisure. Although more people take up pursuits once thought to be the prerogative of the rich such as sailing, fly fishing, climbing, riding and motor racing, and more people see learning as a continuing process, on the other hand there has been a decline in the pursuit of entertainment outside the home such as theatre, cinema and concert-going, and there is probably less entertaining within the home. People no longer inform themselves politically by going to public meetings and themselves taking part in the argument; this information is provided by the television interview and debate, from the comfort of the arm chair. Young peer groups do, however, look for excitement outside the home, often on the football terraces or in the disco, probably because all the family interests cannot be catered for in one evening's viewing, and small families mean that adolescents must go outside to find their coevals.

Whether society is more violent is debatable; it is largely a matter of detection, reporting and labelling. Television news favours the spectacular, hi-jacks and street riots are good visual 'clips', and the labelling of deviant groups can become, as many sociologists have pointed out, a self-fulfilling prophesy.[9] But Victorian London was a very unsafe place; it was often the scene of gang warfare and mugging, and street riots with a death toll have been endemic since the beginning of the industrial revolution. Historically, violence has always occurred when there has been a mixture — in some proportion — of high unemployment, racism and hostility to the police and authority, one, to some extent, leading to the other. Health workers in areas where social unrest is high have a particular duty to be sensitive to its causes, and, no matter what the provocation to avoid being judgemental. Sometimes health workers will find themselves in conflict with regard to their duty to the patient, their duty as a citizen and their own personal values; some of these problems are looked at in Chapter 6.

Immigrants

The fact that England is a multiracial society is hammered home by the media, but this is nothing new, England has accepted many waves of refugees, and in the last 200 years has constantly imported other nationals, particularly for low-paid labour — such as working in mental hospitals.

Some nationals, for example Hungarian refugees, integrate quickly, but others, particularly those whose life style is dominated by their religion often struggle to retain their culture in an alien society, and those who suggest that they should 'adopt the customs of their host country' have surely not seen a small English community in an oriental setting. Health workers dealing with an immigrant population should acquaint themselves with the customs and codes of the nationals with whom they are dealing: for example, the dietary restrictions laid down by the Koran and the codes about family relationships and dress. Sometimes, when dealing with families where children are undernourished because of these restrictions the health worker will need to use great persuasion and tact, and the same applies when dealing with the fasting prescribed by the Jewish Yom Kippur and the Muslim Ramadan. Another difficult problem arises from the uneven syncretisation within families which may lead to conflict. Women, for example, tend to experience cultural shock more than men, and children may cross the divide so quickly that they become alienated from their family. It is important that each group's individual beliefs, provided they do not produce harm to others, their religion and their personal dignity, are respected however alien those beliefs may be to the adviser.

The Alternative Society

While most of the health worker's clientele will have developed 'middle class' values, some will have rebelled against the consumer society. This may include experimenting with mystic religions and through this to oriental concepts of healing. It may involve new attitudes to ecology and to growth, and especially to the industrial growth that has been so much a feature of the last 200 years. For some the better life may be found in communal living and the twentieth century has seen experiments right across the ideological spectrum: the monastic ideal never quite dies. Many people, of course, are disenchanted with traditional medicine which can transplant hearts but not cure the common cold, and there are groups of 'radical midwives', 'radical health visitors' and others who are looking for a new approach to health care.

Life styles that were once regarded as eccentric and outlawed, such as homosexuality, are tolerated in a new light and the same is becoming true of extramarital cohabitation. It is important to remember that the social mores of the mid-twentieth century were not always thus. The Greeks tolerated and, indeed, glorified pederasty, rural mediaeval England expected proof of fertility before marriage and in many periods courtesans had an honoured place. It is likely that mores will change again. It is possible that as contraception becomes more effective and we become more worried about overpopulation and the prospect of unemployment, that we will "regard extra marital cohabitation as unselfish, loving unlimited shared succorance without legal bonds as an example to those toiling in the bonds of matrimony".[10]

The moral problem for the health worker in a time of rapid social and cultural change is how much to condone, how much to tolerate or come to terms with, and where, if anywhere, is the sticking point. Chapters 5 and 6 try to give some help but in the last analysis much depends on the beliefs of the individual worker: for example, Roman Catholics will not condone, or in any way help with abortion, and many people of other religious persuasions, or none, will have scruples about putting schoolgirls on the pill. However, there must be one abiding duty, whatever our personal convictions, and that is to counsel patients and clients against life styles that are a potential danger to health.

Organising the Health Services to Meet New Needs

The administrative framework of the health services is dictated by its historical past, by what is politically expedient and possible, and by the extent of professional pressure. The professions themselves must take some responsibility for the way the services are. The fact that mechanistic medicine had had the greatest resources is largely due to the fact that it has had the most powerful spokesmen and has had the greatest dramatic impact on the public.

As the result of reports in the inter-war period and public pressure for a fairer society, a committee was set up in 1941 to "survey the existing insurance schemes of social and allied services, including workmen's compensation, and to make recommendations". The result was the *Beveridge Report* which provided the basis for the post-war social legislation and was the first attempt by any government to deal with the problem of poverty.

Intrinsic to the plan was the concept of a National Health

Service. However, because the services had grown up to meet different needs in different traditions there were a number of powerful interests that proved difficult to reconcile, and the plan when it came in 1946 was a compromise. The new service was not a revolution, but a taking over of the services as they had evolved at that time and fixing them with legislation. These services had been designed to meet the needs of the early part of the century, but the social changes outlined above were accelerating, and for this reason the structure and its rigidity were even then unsatisfactory.

Apart from this, in order to keep the peace between the vested interests, the services were tripartite (Figure 5). The hospitals were under the Hospitals Division whose powers were delegated to Regional Hospital Boards who in turn devolved responsibility for the personal health and environmental health services with the chief officer remaining the Medical Officer of Health. Health visitors and school nurses were employed directly, and district nurses and midwives were either employed directly or through an agency like the Queen's Institute of District Nursing. Thus, the curative and preventive services were firmly put asunder.

The general practitioners had been largely against the proposed legislation and insisted in remaining 'independent practitioners' with a contract for service (not of service) and being paid on a per capita basis. The family practitioner, therefore, had little contact with either the hospital or the preventive services and for this reason the skills of the health visitors and district nurses were underused.

The division meant that the three arms of the service could be dealing with the same patient—and possibly be giving conflicting advice—and as the needs of the population changed so the disadvantages of the structure grew more obvious. There were, for example, more elderly sick people suffering from degenerative changes and a multiplicity of problems that involved all the services and demanded cooperation and coordination between them. In some cases there were gaps in the service, such as chiropody, which no one supplied; in other cases there were overlaps, for example, antenatal care might well be supplied by all three services.

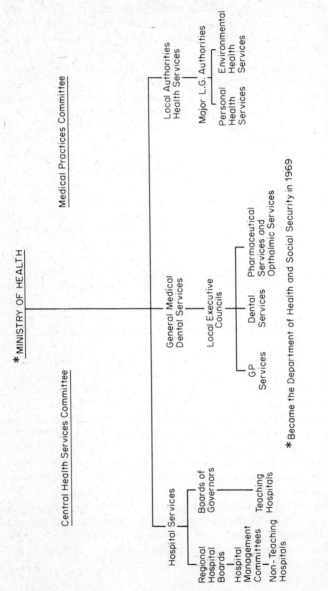

Figure 5. The structure of the National Health Service from 1948 to 1974. (Reproduced from McKeown T. & Low C. R. 1966 *Introduction to Social Medicine*. Oxford: Blackwell Scientific Publications)

* Became the Department of Health and Social Security in 1969

There had been criticism of the structure since the inception of the service, but a number of reports and research studies including *Home from Hospital*[5] and *Care in the Balance*[11] drew attention to the fact that patients were neglected not because the services were not there but because they were divided and did not communicate with one another. This is a good example of the importance of professional pressure effecting change to meet new needs. At the same time, more adventurous spirits in the community were embarking on experiments to make the delivery of care more effective by 'attaching' some health visitors and district nurses to selected group practices. 'Attachment' had its critics but in 1963 it received an impetus from the Committee on the *Future Scope of General Practice* under the chairmanship of Dr Annis Gillie which recommended that this practice be extended and put forward the concept of the *Primary Care Team*. Although such cooperation has been generally beneficial both to patients and to the job satisfaction of the members of the team it has brought problems of accountability which have been exacerbated by subsequent changes in the senior nursing structure and the employing authority of nurses. The issue has been further confused in some cases by the family practitioners privately employing 'practice nurses' over whom the doctor does have a structural authority and who are not responsible to a nursing officer.

In 1968 the *Mayston Report* which followed the Salmon Report on the Senior Nursing Structure in Hospitals, tried to rationalise the nursing structure in the community nursing service to match the structure of the *health service at that time*. The report recommended that all nursing staff, whatever their speciality, should be responsible to their employing authority (i.e. local authority) through a Chief Nursing Officer. In most authorities the report was implemented and although it, like the Salmon Report, was soon to be overshadowed by the reorganisation of the health services in 1974, it did help to clarify the line of accountability and it made the dovetailing of the nursing service easier than it would otherwise have been.

However, the situation was further confused by the position of the social services. Before 1970 the Public Health Services of the Local Authorities included the welfare services, and the same department that employed the health visitors also employed social workers, so that, although the curative and preventive health services had been divorced in 1948, health and welfare were still cohabiting and usually under the same roof. While this had its advantages, the social workers were vociferous about the disadvantages, and the result was the *Seebohm Committee* which issued a report in 1968 recommending that the social services should have a separate department under their own Director. While both departments were answerable to the same authority and covered the same areas this was no great barrier.

But the local authorities themselves were about to change. In 1970 the new government finally rejected the proposals of the Royal Commission on Local Government and brought in its own *Local Government Act* 1974 which provided for a two-tier system with the major authorities based on the old countries with some newly created ones and six metropolitan areas. The newly formed *Department of Social Services* was now based in the major authority. Meanwhile there had been two green papers on the unification of the health services, but now a new difficulty arose; if there was to be easy communication between the health and social services, workers should know one another and, it was argued, the boundaries of the areas they covered should be coterminous. This was a major factor in dictating the structure of the reorganised health services and of the NHS *(Reorganisation) Act 1974.*

The Act sought to achieve unification by bringing the personal health services under the same authority that administered the hospitals. Now district nurses, health visitors and school nurses were the employees of the Area Health Authority and were responsible to them through a hierarchy of nursing officers. As the Royal Commission on Local Government had forecast earlier, the county areas—with which the Area Health Authorities were coterminous, were too large for day-to-day administrators and much of the responsibility had to be developed on to 'Districts'. The lines of communication and the chain of command lengthened. This probably had only a marginal effect of nurses and health visitors working in Primary Care teams, but what did effect them was their separation from the social services. Since most of the cases of child abuse that have ended in tragedy relate to a failure in communication between the health and the social services this separation is of some importance. Moreover, the reorganisation of 1974 did nothing to change the relationship of the Family Practitioner Service to the rest of the health service—it remained largely independent and did not operate within the ordinary cash limits.

The 'Patients First' Reorganisation 1982

As a result of the recommendations of *The Royal Commission on the National Health Service* in 1979, the government produced a document entitled *Patients First* which concerned the administration of the service, and which recommended certain changes in the structure of the health service as set up in 1974. These changes are now being implemented. District Health Authorities now replace Area Health Authorities with the responsibility for day-to-day administration broken down into units (Figure 6). However, the new organisation still leaves a number of important problems untouched. For example, it does not deal with the division between the health and social services whose operational areas are now even less likely to be coterminous, little so far has been done to bring the family practitioners effectively within the ambit of the District Authority, and it does nothing to alter the balance of priorities between the arms of the service or the geographical areas. Moreover, although the Community Health Councils have been saved from extinction, there are no signs that the services have the means to make themselves more sensitive to the needs of the average citizen. District nurses and health visitors have now had their employing authority changed three times in eight years and senior nurses in all branches of the service have spent a decade in uncertainty. Since continual change has an effect on morale and efficiency it is worth pondering on the chain of events outlined in this chapter, how they led to a reorganisation of the service, and why, at each stage, reorganisation was implemented in the manner it was, and indeed, why the services were tripartite in the first place. In history things usually happen the way they do because the events, resources and attitudes of the time made that particular course inevitable. It is perhaps worth asking what

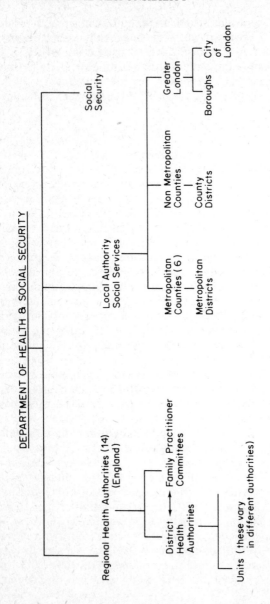

Figure 6. The structure of the DHSS, local government and the National Health Service

have been the attitudes of the health professions to the national health service? Would more professional responsibility towards the perceived needs for health care, rather than the needs for professional status, have avoided some of the pitfalls?

References

1 McKeown T. & Brown R. G. (1969) Interpretation of the rise of the population in England and Wales. *Cent. Afr. J. Med.* Also New Cambridge Modern History, Ch. 8

2 Hobsbawn E. J. (1965) The standard of living during the industrial revolution. *Economic History Review*, **16**, August

3 DHSS (1978) *The Elderly at Home.* London: HMSO

4 Central Statistical Office (1980) Employment statistics. *Social Trends 11*, London: HMSO

5 Skeet M. (1974) *Home from Hospital.* London: Macmillan

6 Rein M. (1970) Problems in the definition and measurement of poverty. In Townsend P. *The Concept of Poverty.* London: William Heinemann

7 Berthoud R. G. (1976) *The Disadvantage of Inequality.* London: Macdonald & James

8 Brown M. & Madge N. (1982) *Despite the Welfare State.* London: William Heinemann

9 Goffman E. (1970) *Stigma: Notes on the Management of Spoiled Identity.* Harmondsworth: Penguin Books

10 Clough N. (1982) Eccentricity. *Nursing Times*, February 14, 274

11 Hockey L. (1968) *Care in the Balance.* London: Queen's Institute of District Nursing

Chapter 3

The Changing Role of the Nurse

The main social changes in society and the new health needs these have created were described in Chapter 2; this chapter looks at the way the nursing services have developed to meet these needs and the professional responsibilities such changes have entailed.

Meeting the New Needs

From the nursing point of view the most obvious change is the age structure of the population. Reading the letters home written by Mary Cadbury in 1879 about her experiences in St Thomas's hospital, and as a district nurse at the new Metropolitan & National Nursing Association, one is struck by the fact that her cases are mostly children and young adolescents; on the district they are often in miserable homes and are dying of such complaints as bronchitis, scarlet fever and diphtheria.[1] Today, children's hospitals deal mainly with investigations and esoteric illness, and there are few children in hospital wards, while the district nurse now rarely has a child on her case load. The nursing problems met with, the skills required, and the psychology in caring for the elderly are very different from those required when nursing young children. A simple practical problem is the weight of the patients concerned. It was one thing for the Victorian nurse, suffering as she frequently was from 'debility' or 'weak ankles', to lift children, it is another thing to lift heavy, inert, elderly patients, and it is significant that as the case load has become literally heavier so nurses have had a higher incidence of 'bad backs' until it is almost an occupational hazard. Mary Cadbury and her contemporaries, on the other hand, suffered from sore throats and scarlet fever which they caught from their young patients, and sometimes from typhoid and typhus which is a testimony to the poor sanitation of the houses and, sad to relate, the hospitals in which they worked.

Demographic change has affected the work of the health visitor. With her roots in the early Visiting Societies of the mid nineteenth century, the first 'health missioners' were all-purpose health educators teaching healthy living to the whole family, but by the end of the century reports and subsequent legislation concentrated mainly on the health of children and the health visitor soon became mainly concerned with the health of mothers and infant welfare. The notification of births to the Medical Officer of Health legitimated the health visitor's work in this respect, and mothers, babies and toddlers took precedence over all else even when the problems of malnutrition had been replaced by overfeeding. The demographic transition means that health visitors need to return to their original role. But the needs of the beginning of the century are still there; marriage is, or has been, earlier and childbearing sooner, and mothers still need advice. Indeed, in spite of improved education, the daughter of a small family is less likely to know about the practical problems of motherhood than did her great-grandmother who was possibly one of eight children. However, clients now expect more and a higher standard, there is more to be known, and no one person can be an expert in all fields. Although it is important to limit the number of visitors to the home and not to destroy the unique relationship between the family and their particular health visitor, specialist help must be accepted, good examples being the service offered by the Community Psychiatric Nurse and specialised help with handicapped children. It is part of continuing professional responsibility to estimate critically when specialities are needed for the profession and to take responsibility for how these are developed and the training provided (see The Development of Nursing Specialities below).

Housing

How people live often effects their need for institutional care. All too often the hospitals of today are used for the charities of yesterday and for "patients who are socially deprived and badly housed, who are not evidence of the need for a hospital bed but of the failure in the social and economic programme".[2] These words were written 19 years ago but they are still largely true; elderly patients cannot be discharged because their home is not suitable, or they have no available relatives or other carers, and there is no alternative home or hostel in the community. The fact that the hospital bed now costs upwards of £100 a day[3] should concentrate the minds of planners, and the Treasury, because there is little hope of the hospital service budget being maintained—let alone reduced, unless there are alternatives in the community to hospital care.

Housing patterns and new life styles make a difference to the way district nurses and health visitors organise their work. There is, for example, the problem of a new housing estate where no one seems to be at home between 9 am and 5 pm and the nurse perforce must make her visits in the evening, along with the canvassers, flag sellers and commercial travellers.

The early health visitors contended with the sanitary conditions in the back-to-back houses, many with the W.C. outside, and tenement flats with the only water tap on the stairs. But the new psychological problems created by the vast concrete and glass blocks are such that even the architects admit that they have created more problems than they have solved, and sociologists are re-appraising the worth of the old life style that centred on nineteenth-century urban, industrial dwellings.

For these reasons, early nursing education programmes concentrated on hygiene and this subject figures largely in examination papers both as a practical subject and as elementary science, which included a certain amount of chemistry and physics. This emphasis on cleanliness and hygiene sprang largely from the fact that the planners of the early courses, including, of course, Miss Nightingale herself, adhered firmly to the miasma theory, and they thought that disease was primarily due to dirt and poor ventilation; thus, in many ways they taught the right thing for the wrong reason. Of course it was ultimately necessary to know the right reason, and once the right reason is known there is no need to be so fanatical on the subject. While the need to teach domestic hygiene still remains—and it is by no means always good—the health visitor of today must understand more about the sociology of modern living and the psychology of her clients. It is, however, worth reflecting that the deprived child with behaviour problems may also be miserable because of the irritation of head lice.

The Economy

The main contributing factor to the mantle of disease across the world is insufficient, or the wrong kind of, food, and poor environmental conditions. The western industrial nations have, however, tended to replace the diseases of poverty with the diseases of affluence which include alcoholism, accidents from sport and 'leisure' pursuits, drug addiction and ischaemic heart disease due to tension and high-powered living. Nevertheless, pockets of poverty do remain, particularly among immigrants and old people, who either do not know their rights or for reasons of pride or tradition do not take them up. Once again it is Social Class V that suffers most; pensioners from Class I and II not only have better pensions, more assets and probably a better chance of continuing some part-time earning, they also know their entitlements and accept them.

In 1900 the clients and patients may have been absolutely poor, but it was a fairly stable poverty; 23/- a week (115p) fed the average family and the budget and wages remained the same year after year.[4] During the 1930s the cost of living actually went down because high unemployment meant that it was a buyer's market. Between 1938–1947 the cost of living rose by 100 points, and between 1970 and 1980 by 300 points. The pound worth 100p at the close of the Second World War is now worth about 10p.[5] Rapid inflation not only undermines the currency, it destroys faith in institutions and it creates anxieties in a way that stable poverty does not; this is particularly true for old people living on fixed incomes who can remember when bread was 4d (about 1½p) a loaf, and anxiety is a contributing factor in many of the cases presenting themselves at the doctor's surgery.

Therefore nurses, both in hospital and in the community are dealing not only with a different age group but with a different mantle of disease, for which they require a different preparation. Furthermore, although the need for health education is as great as ever it was, it must now be directed at a different target. Education to combat the destruction of health caused by tension, alcoholism, smoking, drug taking or simply teenagers tearing round the block on fast motorbikes, is infinitely more difficult and needs more subtlety than that required for handing out tracts or hygiene and carbolic soup. Miss Nightingale saw all nurses as sanitary missioners, not only giving advice, but by precept and example—hence all those clean aprons; today, this remains part of our professional responsibility, and in one respect at least, namely that of smoking, (48 per cent of hospital nurses still smoke), they are doing less well than their medical colleagues.

The Structure of the Services

The National Health Service has brought about an important change inasmuch as it is a universal service for all classes of the community. This new universality is important in looking at the changed role of the nurse. The early reformed nurses were forbidden to go into private practice because the needs of the poor were so overwhelming, the poor expected little and for the most part were suitably grateful. Today, patients know more and expect more information: on the whole they remain grateful, but nurses now have a responsibility to be sensitive to the needs, and level of intelligence and social habits, of all groups in society, and this requires more versatility than just being good and compassionate with the sick poor.

Apart from this, changes within the structure of the service itself affect the role of the nurse. One example is the attachment of health visitors and district nurses to group practice. District nurses are now much more likely to work in cooperation with family doctors and to be asked to undertake primary assessment, and, with early discharge from hospital, to find themselves responsible for ever more complicated treatment and advanced techniques, carrying around in the back of the car equipment once reserved for special units in hospitals. The health visitor, on the other hand, has come firmly within the ambit of the primary health care team rather than in the social services, and this has altered her nearest colleagues and the planning of her work; her clients are now more scattered and no longer can she hope—with luck—to do all the toddlers in Coronation Street in one day. Attachment had its advantages, but one of the disadvantages is finding enough time for primary prevention—and there is still plenty to be done.

Changing Training and Education to Meet These New Responsibilities

The Hospital Nurse

The aim of the early reformed nursing in the mid-nineteenth century which soon took hold in many large general hospitals, was that it should be essentially practical and based on ward teaching. But who would, or should, teach the new probationers? The only people available were the old-style nurses who the reformers so often affected to despise, and who in any case, as the Nightingale Fund found out, often had not the time. There was, of course, the possibility of the doctors but the new regime had built its Empire by wresting the control of nurses from the doctors, and they were mostly hostile. In 1880 the British Medical Journal carried an article which stated that "there should be sufficient trained nurses to carry out the orders of the doctors to whom they should look, and *to whom alone they should look for orders and guidance.*"[6] Another possibility was the introduction of better-educated recruits as 'training sisters' and a Home Sister—who was virtually a nurse tutor—but of course the better educated wanted, and could take, more theory. In spite of these innovations it is significant that the doctors' lectures continued to give detailed information about nursing practice such as the making of poultices and the prevention of bed sores.[7] But as medicine became more scientific some of the hostility fell away and the British Medical Journal, in a Machiavellian moment, pointed out that "the doctors gave the lectures and they could control what was taught." If the examinations were anything to go by they taught what they themselves knew best, anatomy, physiology, chemistry and physics. Nursing was caught on the horns of a dilemma; to remain practical and appeal as an occupation to a motivated working class—and stay clear of the doctors—or to advertise itself as 'scientific' and appeal to the better educated who would, of course, absorb more and more of what the doctors could teach. In the end, of course, it vacillated, but the more prestigious schools were those with the most lectures and the most difficult examination questions on the medical model. By 1907 there are questions about the heart sounds and how they are produced and about the nervous system and the testing of various reflexes.[8] The doctors had clearly given up keeping the new nurses at bay and were training them as their assistants.

"Doctors changed their relationship with their patients based on the doctor's response to the signs and symptoms of the disease, this made it necessary to carry out new kinds of continuous and detailed investigations of the course of diseases . . . As the doctors developed the thermometer and the sphygmonameter so these were entrusted to nurses while the doctors passed to more sophisticated work".[9] The nurses in their turn shuffled off some of those practical tasks to other grades. By the early years of the twentieth century nurses were justifying their clamour for status and registration by the fact that they carried out the doctor's orders and were his assistants. For all the vaunted benefits of registration there seems little change in the curriculum and in the way knowledge was tested. A Final State examination paper in 1930, which incidentally included a question on the application of leeches, reads much like the paper of 1907 referred to earlier. There was, of course, a certain amount of levelling up—more nurses were able to describe the heart sounds—and while the health needs of the population were mainly episodic and acute there was some justification for the medical model emphasis. After all, the nursing of pneumonia did depend on an understanding of the physiological changes, accurate measuring and acute observation. However, soon this represented only a small part of the total needs for nursing care. It is arguable whether the statutory control of the basic nurse training allowed it to be flexible enough to adapt the programme quickly. Statutory control was, of course, linked with the fact that it was financially advantageous to the hospitals and the government for probationers to meet the service needs of the hospital wards, therefore, ipso facto, training was mainly about meeting those needs. But it is a hallmark of a profession that it is responsible for its own education programme and the question to be asked is, how well has nursing exercised that responsibility, and how is it going to exercise it in the future?

The District Nurse

People have always been nursed at home, usually by relatives, friends or servants, but sometimes by those with a special vocation for helping the sick such as the Vincentian Sisters of Mercy. Modern district nursing is an extension of the reformed nursing system with part of the money from the Nightingale Fund being used to help the Metropolitan & National Nursing Association in Bloomsbury Square. This long and rigorous training based on the hospital and the district, and which produced its own trained nursing superintendents, became the basis of training favoured by the Queen Victoria's Jubilee Institute for Nurses when it came into being in 1887. The training required for district nurses was longer and more exacting than that required for a hospital nurse and it is interesting to note that the first trainees were all 'specials' that is to say 'lady probationers' although several were in fact 'free specials'.[10] The Queen's nurses were held in high regard, and although in fact they were never responsible for all the home nursing, they set the standard for emulation.

In 1936 the *Midwives Act*, in an attempt to improve the maternal mortality rates, required all local authorities to employ salaried midwives and many did this through the agency of the Queen's Institute. In rural areas many nurses were employed who were triply trained. However, more and more people were using the hospitals, and insurance schemes of various kinds enabled more people to use the doctor's surgery, therefore, the district nurse tended to lose her place as the surrogate doctor, and to be mainly concerned with the long-term, housebound, chronic sick. Nor did the coming of the National Health Service help matters; district nurses were now further divided from their colleagues because of the structure of the service, and the image of the district nurse as only capable of attending to the routine needs of the long-term sick became a self-fulfilling prophesy at a time when the health needs of the population were crying out for a wider range of nursing skills for patients at home.

In 1959 a Panel of Assessors was set up to advise the Ministry of Health. In an attempt to gain more 'home nurses' quickly, the training period was reduced to four months and, in spite of protests from the profession, the government insisted on using the *National Certificate* which had no educational status and was simply granted by employing authorities. Although for a time the Queen's Institute carried on providing its own certificate, after 1968 it ceased to be a training body. Meanwhile, research studies carried out by the Institute including *Feeling the Pulse* (1966) and *Care in the Balance* (1968) showed the extravagent waste on the part of hospitals who recalled patients unnecessarily, and the fact that the family practitioners failed to use the expertise of the district nurse and tried to do themselves tasks that would have been better done by the nurse. District nurses themselves, aware that they were not being fully used, clamoured to have their training put on a comparable basis with that of the health visitor. There were considerable grounds for supporting their claim. The cost of the hospital bed was rising dramatically and patients were being discharged to complete their treatment at home earlier. The age structure of the population was changing and there were more sick in the community with fewer relatives to care for them, and more people lived alone. Apart from the enormous cost of hospital care, research had shown the deleterious effects of a stay in hospital: 'home is best' was again fashionable.

In 1970 *The Committee on Nurse Education* under the chairmanship of Professor Asa Briggs (later Lord Briggs) recommended a single Training Council for all branches of nursing; now it seemed possible that district nursing would again be on a parity with other post-basic courses. However, the Training Councils to be displaced by the new Central Council feared, with some justification when they looked at the record for basic training, that the programmes likely to be offered by the new Council would be inferior to those they had already achieved, and they therefore demanded—and eventually received—a promise of separate committees in the new structure. This left the district nurses in the same anomalous position. In 1979 the *Panel of Assessors* was reconstituted and its membership enlarged and, together with district nurses themselves, they lobbied to have their own committee and premises under the aegis of the new *United Kingdom Central Council for Nursing, Midwifery and Health Visiting*. Eventually a new curriculum based on the nursing process and the up-to-date needs of the district nurse as a member of the primary care team, came into force in 1981, and this is now mandatory before anyone can use the title 'district nurse'.

The story of district nursing since the National Health Service is a triumph of professional responsibility over bureaucracy. It was cheaper, in the short term, to have merely a perfunctory training for district nurse and this is what successive Ministries had advocated, but district nurses and their more enlightened colleagues knew better, and persisted, sometimes against great odds, that they be given a training that fitted them to meet the needs of their patients today.

Health Visitors

Fredrick Verney, who was largely responsible for the experimental training of health visitors in Buckinghamshire, said "A health visitor in not a nurse and does not pretend to be one."[11] His aunt, Florence Nightingale, had said earlier "I use the term nursing for want of a better"[12] and she herself saw nursing as something wider than carrying out the doctor's orders. There is still confusion about the proper task of the nurse and much print has been expended on whether the health visitor should be a nurse, but until the first is settled the later is really superfluous. The early concept of a 'health visitor' grew out of the work of the people used by the various Visiting societies that tended to spring up after the *Health of Towns Commission* in 1844: later it was conceded that they would be more effective if they were trained. It was Miss Nightingale's idea that if such people were trained they would form a back-up service for the work of the new district nurses in which she was greatly interested. Since disease was due to 'miasma', once sanitation was improved and people were taught to be clean and to ventilate their houses, then they could look to the day when there would be "only nurses to the well". If that prognostication appears naïve, it should be compared with that made by the planners of the National Health Service that once the backlog of ill health was treated, the costs would fall.

The idea of health visiting appealed to numbers of educated women who wanted a career in health care but who were daunted by the publicised discipline required for nurse training and the new power of the matron to dismiss without question. The first health visitors included sanitary officers, university graduates and women doctors whom, one suspects, were unable to get a post in traditional medicine because the doors were closed against them by their male colleagues. In 1907 both Bedford and Battersea Colleges were offering courses for candidates without nursing qualifications, thus providing a heritage of training within higher education which has always marked off health visiting from other post-basic nursing education.

As pointed out earlier, concern about the health of children and the passing of the *Notification of Births Act* 1907 caused health visitors to focus on the health of mothers and babies, and nurses and midwives looking for an escape from the discipline and the stifling atmosphere of hospital nursing soon outnumbered all other applicants. By 1918 half the applicants were nurses and most of them had more than one nursing qualification. When the first Ministry of Health came into being in 1919 there were three methods of entry:

> a one-year basic course for a person already qualified as a nurse, that is, after 1925, a State-registered general nurse;
> a different one-year training for a person already a university graduate; and
> a two-year training (later extended by six months) for non-graduates who were not nurses.

Many people see these three methods of entry as providing a basis for a unified medico-social profession and its abandonment as a lost opportunity. With hindsight this may appear so, but given the attitudes and needs of the day some fragmentation was probably historically inevitable. In 1925 a new training was devised and the Royal Sanitary Institute selected as an examining body—there was no suggestion that there should be any connection with the General Nursing Council. After this date all entrants were required to have a training in midwifery which, incidentally, ensured that they were women.

With a continuing high infant mortality rate and poor child health during the years of unemployment in the 1930s this training sufficed, but with the changed circumstances after the Second World War the question arose: Was this training suitable to meet the new needs? By 1950 the infant mortality rate was down to 28 per 1000, diphtheria and other bacterial diseases were fast disappearing and, paradoxically, because of rationing, evacuation and enforced attention to health education in the war, children were better cared for and healthier than they had ever been. But the health visitor was debarred from expanding her role to the whole family because she was isolated both from the general practitioners and her colleagues in hospital—a further example of the way the structure of the service can dictate what nurses do. The situation was made worse by the new impetus to techniques in hospitals and the fact that there was little or nothing about preventive medicine in the basic courses for nurses or doctors.

The health visitor had duties as a school nurse and also to fostered children under the *Child Life Protection Acts 1908*, and to mentally handicapped children cared for at home, but, with the coming of the National Health Service the former was less highly regarded (see below) and the latter was transferred to the Children's Officers after the setting up of Children's Departments following the *Curtis Report* in 1946. Health visitors themselves, concerned at the failure to use their skills, called for an enquiry through their professional organisations. In 1953 a working party under the chairmanship of Sir Wilson Jameson was set up "To advise on the proper field of recruitment and training of health visitors in the National Health Service and the School Health Service". The report issued in 1956 emphasised that the health visitor had "the opportunity to act as a common point of reference and a source of standard information and that the health visitor could be in a real sense a general purpose family visitor."[13]

At the same time a similar working party under the chairmanship of Miss Younghusband made recommendations about the training of social workers who had a variety of different trainings and whose work often overlapped with that of the health visitor. The result of these two reports was that in 1962 the *Health Visitor and Social Worker Training Act* set up a Council for the Education and Training of Health Visitors (CETHV) and a Council for Training Social Workers, with a chairman and some members in common which, it was hoped, would prevent overlapping. The new Council replaced the Royal Society for Health (formerly the Royal Sanitary Institute) as the examining body and issued a new curriculum and set out to provide a more holistic education for health visitors. These events are important because, as already shown, this independent and more academic education became the paradigm that the planners of other post-basic courses wished to emulate, and was the main reason why they regarded a new Central Council, thought to favour apprenticeship methods, with some suspicion.

To a large extent the two training councils cleared up the boundary disputes as to who should be trained for what, and now that the health visitors work within the Health Service while the social workers are with the Social Services Departments of the local authority the distinction is more clear. On the other hand, the two services whose tasks were often complementary, have lost the close touch they had with one another in the days when the both worked with the Medical Officer of Health. There are losses as well as gains.

Like their district nursing colleagues, health visitors have had to fight constantly for recognition and for a training to enable them to match the needs they have to face. Like the district nurses they lost out in the post war years but have recently regained their professional status, not because of policy from above, but by their own dogged determination and professional sense. It is perhaps to be expected that health visitors who are, literally, paid to be articulate and to convince people should be convincing in their own cause.

School Nurses

Although demographic change has made little obvious difference to the work of school nurses, their work perhaps more than that of other groups has altered as the result of social change.

School nurses were supplied by voluntary bodies at the end of the nineteenth century but their real legitimacy came with the *Education (Administrative Provisions) Act 1907.* Arrangements to meet the needs of this Act were not uniform; some authorities used their health visitors to cover the service, others thought it outrageously socialist and a usurpation of the rights of parents and did little. The Public Health Section of the College of Nursing when it was formed argued that health visitors should perform the service because they would be able to follow through children in their areas from the womb to work, and argument which lost its force with attachment to group practices and the frequent reorganisation of schools. Moreover, in large cities large schools needed a separate and highly concentrated service and some authorities developed a distinct school nursing service for which training was often offered on an ad hoc basis.

With the coming of the National Health Service, central and local government, wishing to save money, maintained that a school health service was an unnecessary luxury. Children were healthier and with their short hair and better standards of hygiene, scabies, ringworm and head lice were a thing of the past, and in any event they were able to visit their own family doctor and have treatment free of charge. The policy of the Ministry of Health was to cease to require a specific number of checks and to reduce the whole service, a situation not conducive to the promotion of a training for the school nurse.

But for those working in the school health service the position was not quite as the Ministry foretold. Physically healthier children produced more problems, they matured earlier and had sexual and emotional problems undreamed of in the under-nourished children of the past. Children stayed at school until they were 16 years old, some were non-academic and bored, other were pushed by an examination system in which a whole life can depend on A-level results. Both groups took solace in drink or drugs—with fashions running in cycles. Until recently an affluent society had provided pocket money to buy cigarettes and smoking at school had become more common—this is more alarming now the results in terms of cancer are known. Divorce was higher and more children come from broken homes, and while the administrators were running down the service, the problems of children and immigrant groups in the inner cities were mounting. The school nurse now faces problems unthought of by her predecessors. The old scourges of scabies and lice have reappeared, there are about 5 000 known pregnancies a year in girls under 16 years old, the majority of which end in abortion with all the trauma and emotional consequences that this entails. At the same time the Royal Commission on the Health Service pointed to the quite appalling amount of dental decay in school children in some areas of the country and the lack of any meaningful preventive dental service. With violence being perpetuated by younger age groups there is the problem of its causes, how such behaviour can be prevented and, when not prevented, how it should be dealt with subsequently. With young children terrorising mature and seasoned teachers and the burning of school property it is idle to suggest there is now no need for a counselling service. Dealing with these problems calls for social skills and a sophisticated training very different from those needs by school nurses when they had only to persuade parents and pupils to use soap and water.

Furthermore, both the Court Report (1976) and the Warnock Report (1978) point to new responsibilities for the school nurse. The Court Committee suggested that each school should have a specially nominated school doctor and a nurse trained in educational medicine who would have enough time to know the pupils and the teachers and who would visit and counsel on a regular basis. The Warnock Report tackled the problem of the growing number of handicapped children resulting from the higher survival rate and recommended that children should be assessed according to their needs and not according to the category of their handicap, that there should be no minimum age at which education should begin, and that, as far as possible, education should take place in ordinary schools. The report has bccn accepted and the *Education Act 1981*, when it comes into force, will have implications for school nurses. The school nurse will be called upon to help with the assessments of such children and her observations and recommendations may well be vital to their careers.

Meeting the requirements of the Act and of the new social, health and emotional problems outlined above, calls for a different preparation for school nurses, and a training based on the service needs of a general hospital is certainly not suitable. School nurses are aware of their needs and, like their colleagues the district nurses and the health visitors before them, are asking for a training to fit them to meet the needs of the school children of the future.

Other Nursing Specialities

There are two groups of patients and clients who may justify the use of a specialist nurse. One is where a different basic training is required, as in psychiatric nursing; the other is where the nursing problem itself is particularly difficult, as in oncology nursing, stoma care or terminal care, or where it is rare, as in ophthalmic nursing, so that no one 'general' nurse can be expected to have all the expertise. In some instances however, the specialist nurse, as in the case of those advising on terminal care nursing, may eventually prove a leaven to the whole.

The preparation for the first group is in the hands of the statutory body. Over the years these trainings have changed to meet new needs, but whether fast enough is a matter of opinion.

It is the second group that is of particular interest in terms of professional responsibility. The profession has not only a duty to define the specialisms that are needed—and sometimes more important, not needed—it must also develop an educational programme to prepare suitable students, and make sufficient and convincing representations to the government and other bodies such as the King's Fund, to procure the money to fund such courses. In this respect, in the last decade or so, The *Joint Board of Clinical Nursing Studies* has been able to run a number of courses that have been a response to professional pressure to meet what professional opinion has seen as a need.

New Ways of Delivering Health Care

It is the responsibility of the profession itself to decide how best care can be delivered to meet the needs of any particular society at any particular time.

The early reformers of nursing were in a quandary whether nursing should be practical and learnt on the ward, or theoretical and partly learnt elsewhere. For the last hundred years there has been an uneasy compromise. Although the early probationers recruited by the Nightingale Fund were to some extent supernumerary there was soon an argument about what was training and what was service. Miss Nightingale wrote across the diaries which recorded the washing of utensils *"This is not training*, this is *hospital work"*, but in vain. As the costs rose and the Fund's proportional contribution grew less so 'hospital work' predominated.

This has had a number of consequences including the fact that general training — the basis on which all other post-basic training must be built — has been in the acute general hospital and is hospital-task orientated. Also, it has confused the issue about accountability because the trainee nurse has seen herself as an employee and as there to carry out the doctor's orders, but not to initiate care herself. Nursing has been seen as a series of jobs to be done — usually as quickly as possible.

Fortunately nursing research, and the new health needs of society, are forcing a different approach to the whole philosophy of nursing care and what it is about: one outcome of this new thinking is the nursing process. A detailed description of the cycle of assessment, planning, implementation and evaluation that make up the nursing process and the philosophy behind it are outside the scope of this book; it is, however, important to stress that an open mind, a willingness to believe that change is possible, and a continual awareness of research findings and the light these throw on current practice is the hall mark of the professional attitude.

Looked at historically, nursing education in the realms of post-basic nursing would appear to have adapted more readily to meet new needs than the training provided by the foundation course. But the foundation block is vital not only in the knowledge it supplies but in the attitudes it encourages. How, and whether, the foundation course changes is a matter for the profession.

References

1 Cadbury M. Letters held by GLRO.HI/ST/NTS/Y16/1
2 Kemp R. (1964) The golden bed. *Lancet*, **ii**, 7386.
3 Office of Health Economics (1980) *Compendium of Health Statistics*. London: OHE
4 Marwick A. (1965) *The Deluge*. London: Macmillan, p.24
5 Registrar General (1980) *Annual Digest of Statistics*. London: HMSO
6 Bradley S. M. (1980) Letter. *Br. Med. J.*, April 14
7 Croft J. (1874) *Notes of Lectures, Lecture 26*. London: Blades & Blades
8 Examination papers, London. GLRO.HI/ST/NTS/C40
9 Foucault M. C. (1973) *The Birth of a Clinic*. London: Tavistock Press
10 Register of Nurses (B) London. GLRO.HI/ST/NTS/C4
11 Verney F. (1891) *Introduction to Sick Nursing and Health*. Paper written by Miss Florence Nightingale for the Chicago Exhibition 1893
12 Nightingale F. (1859) *Notes on Nursing*. London: Harrison. Reprinted (1952) London: Duckworth
13 Ministry of Health (1956) *Inquiry into Health Visiting (Jameson Report)*. London: HMSO, p.302

Chapter 4

Personal, Legal and Professional Responsibility

It is accepted that when a professional practitioner works independently for a private client he is personally responsible for his professional work. If an architect designs a house and it collapses because of a fault in the design no one will be surprised if he is sued for damages. The same is obvious when a doctor has a contract for service, although it is in some way less clear when there is a contract of service and the practitioner is an employee. However, most people if asked would say that doctors are responsible for what they do or advise and can be held liable at law, hence the emphasis on the importance of doctors belonging to a medical defence society.

Although logically there is no reason why employed nurses should not be held responsible in the same way as employed doctors, there are a number of historical reasons why nurses have seldom been sued by patients, and why they have often not regarded themselves as being independent practitioners and responsible at law for their own acts.

The Development of Professional Responsibility

The historical confusion is bound up with the position of women generally. Even when, in the late nineteenth century, women broke into the ranks of paid non-manual work and into the burgeoning professions, they usually did so in a subordinate role and, except in rare cases, were not expected to exercise independent judgement.[1] The men gave the orders.

In nursing the problem was exacerbated by the confusion over accountability referred to in Chapter 3. Miss Nightingale's aim was not to create a profession for women but to improve the standard of nursing and the care received by the sick. This, she argued, could only be done if nurses were responsible to someone who understood good nursing and who was a trained nurse. Because the Nightingale Fund was prestigious it gradually established that, in most large hospitals at least, nurses should be responsible to a matron or a nurse superintendent. However, no sooner had this revolution occurred than medicine entered the era of the validity of the germ theory of infection. The doctor could now investigate disease with some prospect of cure, and the nurse in the general hospital became the doctor's assistant, carrying out the treatment and investigations he ordered, and in this capacity the nurse was responsible to the doctor. Moreover, doctors were men and nurses were women. The debate over who should control nurses, and have the power to hire, fire and discipline them, continued for a number of years. In a letter in 1872 Henry Bonham Carter, Secretary to the Nightingale Fund, wrote "Doctors are apt to imagine that because they are the proper and only persons to give orders respecting treatment of patients therefore they must have the complete control of the staff". He goes on, with a lawyers logic, to point out that when the doctors had 'control' of nursing staff they had not made a very good job of producing good trained nurses.[2] The debate confused the nurses themselves who, in any event, had had the virtue of obedience instilled into them. If the nurse was there merely to carry out orders there was no reason why she should exercise judgement, and she accepted all too easily the fallacy that the doctor would take the responsibility as he passed his tasks over to her.

The second reason why nurses were seldom sued independently was because they were notoriously poorly paid; furthermore, the voluntary hospitals themselves were unlikely to be the subject of a claim for negligence, because they were always in debt and relied for their funds on voluntary contributions. The ordinary people who carried collecting boxes would not wish to see their money wasted in the courts. Thirdly, before the advent of the legal aid system, the section of the population that used the hospitals and the public health services was remarkably unlitigious, and the mystic of medicine was such that they could easily be blinded by science. As Bernard Shaw said "All professions are a conspiracy against the laity". Finally, until the advent of more powerful drugs, technology and therapy, the nurse's capacity for harm was comparatively limited. Confusion over drachms and ounce signs was not unknown, but except in rare cases, the classic being paraldehyde, it was rarely fatal. A wrong dose of a steroid given intravenously is likely to have more drastic, and less easily reversible, consequences. A slight tear of the perineum is one thing, a mistake in topping up epidural anaesthesia is another.

Today, the situation about the law of tort and the health service is different. Patients and clients use the service as of right, they expect no avoidable harm to occur, they are much better informed about what to expect from the service and more legal and professional advice is available to those who feel aggrieved. Furthermore, since the inception of the National Health Service a body of case law has been built up concerning tort as it applies to the health service; any student of the law reports will need no convincing on that score.

The Position of the Nurse in Law

The nurse has a duty of care towards her patient or client and she is required to be, and to remain, a safe practitioner. The law does not require extraordinary knowledge but that which is compatible with her position, experience and qualifications. A district nurse must, for example, be a safe practitioner in carrying the duties covered in the curriculum of training. The duty to care means that unreasonable risks must not be taken, and the foreseeable consequences must be weighed. These principles apply not only to physical care but also to advice; the wrong advice can lead to harm just as putting a frail patient on a commode without proper precautions can lead to a fall and a fractured femur.

Individually, every practitioner has a duty to keep up to date with matters that affect his or her practice. Having administered a wrong dose of a drug because one's training had been in the imperial measure rather than the metric, it is of little avail to offer this as an excuse in a court of law. However, the law also lays a duty of care in health authorities. The first duty is to provide care for the patients and public under its care, the second is a duty to the staff it employs, and this includes ensuring that they are properly qualified and instructed to carry out care for those in their charge. An authority would be in breach of duty if it employed auxiliaries to give controlled drugs, or if it failed to ensure that staff returning to work after a considerable break were given an adequate in-service training.

The Patients' and Clients' Rights

Patients and clients have certain rights at law. For example, no one may interfere with the body of another person without the consent of that person, and anyone who does so is liable to an action for damages. Secondly, a nurse being in a fiduciary capacity, that is a position of trust, must preserve a patient's confidence unless relieved of that obligation (see Chapter 6). Thirdly, and of particular importance to health workers in the community, the patient has a right to expect that no avoidable harm shall be done to his property or his reputation. If the patient, client or relatives feel that harm has resulted because of negligence they may bring an action for damages. The action will be brought against the person or persons against whom the action is most likely to succeed and this will depend on the advice given to the litigant. What is harm and what is avoidable and who was responsible are matters for the law. However, the law may ask for assistance from an 'expert witness'. For example, if a nurse has lifted an elderly patient out of bed on a hoist and the patient has fallen and sustained injuries, an independent, senior nurse who has experience in such matters may be called to testify whether reasonable precautions were taken, whether the procedure adopted was commensurate with established practice and what is taught, and whether the equipment used was suitable, properly serviced, issued with instructions, and safe. A great responsibility rests on those called to give help in this way.

Claims for Negligence

Even if the claim is made against the employing authority, if a nurse is involved, he or she would be well advised to seek personal advice from her professional organisation. Much has been written about the vicarious responsibility of the employing authority for acts of negligence on the part of its staff and the fact that in the end it is generally the authority who foots the bill, and it is sometimes suggested that professional organisations are making too much of the issue of legal responsibility. When claims are composite this might appear to be the case, but the question is not as simple as that. The legal notes in the *Hospital Year Book* are explicit:

"It appears to be established that a hospital authority, whether public authority, voluntary or commercial, will be vicariously liable for injury caused by the negligence or incompetence of any members of its staff, medical, medical auxiliaries, nursing, domestic or other. It makes no difference whether they work whole time or part time and whether they work under a contract of service or for service. *The negligent person is also liable and the hospital has a right at common law to claim indemnity against that person.*"[3]

But writers who concentrate on the payment of damages, by whom, to whom and for what, obscure other important issues. With a complicated claim in the offing, employing authorities sometimes try to discourage personal defence on the grounds that too many solicitors or professional advisors around tend to play up the importance of the claim and may cause conflict. While it is obviously important to avoid making too much of a trivial claim, it must be remembered that in a composite claim the undefended may bear the brunt of the legal censure; this is particularly true in the case of accidents in the operating theatre where many people were involved, and the parallel could be treatments carried out in the doctor's surgery or the Health Centre—everyone blames someone else. Moreover, the defence of an individual is not necessarily the same as that of the Management, who will naturally maintain that they carried out their duty by having the right staff, in the right numbers and with the right equipment in the right place at the right time. That could be contrary to the defence of the nurse; for example her advocate may claim, and usually with justice, that the nurse in question had to leave the patient in order to attend to others because there were no other staff on duty at that time.

The main point to remember is not the likelihood of the claim for damages but the possibility of being found blameworthy without justification. If a nurse is found to be negligent it is most likely that disciplinary action will be taken against her, if it is serious her name removed from the register. Even if the outcome is not so draconian, being labelled 'negligent' is an unpleasant and unnerving experience—it is emotionally upsetting and many have consequences for the worker's future working relationships.

Nor are nursing officers with managerial functions exempt, although they may not cause avoidable harm themselves, they can be cited as contributing to negligence, for example, by failing to ensure that nursing staff are properly instructed in the use of new equipment or techniques.

Procedure in the Event of a Professional Accident

As soon as it is clear that an accident has taken place that might involve the practitioner—even indirectly, she should get in touch with her professional organisation responsible for arranging personal legal defence. The organisation will probably have an arrangement with insurers who will send a legal representative as soon as possible. From then on the practitioner should be guided by the legal adviser.

A number of problems arise in the interim. The accident must be reported and some authorities have standard rules which must be complied with and factual data should be recorded as soon as possible. Statements should be confined to facts, but no one should be expected to incriminate himself. The authority should be told that the matter is in the hands of the professional organisation and that further statements will be made by the legal adviser. The incident should not be discussed with other members of the staff and on no account should resignation be offered or dismissal accepted.

If a member of the nursing health care team is called to give evidence about an accident, this should be confined to factual and accurate information without digression into opinion, irrelevant matter of supposition.

Fear of litigation is a poor basis for good practice, and in spite of the foregoing, serious professional negligence is comparatively rare. However, accidents can happen, even apparently when every precaution has been taken, as every car driver knows. When they do happen they bring misery and often damaging anxiety which in itself may lead to injudicious comment. On such occasions there is no substitute for independent personal advice and even an independent shoulder on which to weep.

Remaining a Safe Practitioner

In a rapidly changing service, in which technological, medical and pharmaceutical methods of treatment advance at a bewildering rate, how can the average practitioner remain safe?

Clarity about Accountability

In the last 20 years the issue of accountability has been confused by the changes in the employing authority referred to in Chapter 2. This confusion has been confounded by changes in the nursing command structure brought about by the implementation of the Salmon and Mayston Reports, the reorganisation of the health service in 1974 and again in 1982 and in the case of the primary health care team the situation is complicated by the policy of group attachment. Nurses in middle management may find that the title of their nursing superior has changed five times in 16 years. One of the criticisms of the Royal Commission on the Health Service was that the elongated chain of command delayed decision making and there was confusion about responsibility, accountability and what was meant by 'monitoring'. It is important that each professional worker has a contract of service which sets out clearly to whom he or she is accountable.

The other problem for the primary health care team is that different members are accountable to different authorities. The nurse members of the team are responsible to the District Health

Authority usually through the Community Services Nursing Officer, although different districts have different units. The social workers are accountable to the Director of Social Services in the local authority, in an office possibly geographically remote. The doctors are responsible to the Family Practitioner Committee, and the practice nurse, receptionist and practice manager—if these are employed—are directly accountable to the doctors. In spite of the confusion this entails, most groups find a modus vivendi and accept one another's expertise as the situation demands. Good team personal relationships can largely overcome the structural conflicts, and if difficulties do arise nursing officers then have a responsibility to act as arbitrators.

'arrangement between people who agree to differ'

Confidence in Ability to Undertake Tasks

Practitioners should not accept responsibility for tasks they do not feel safe to undertake. This prohibition is included in the International Code of Nursing Ethics[4] but is not always put into practice. Unfortunately, medicine and nursing set much store by the ability to perform technical tasks and this in nursing, with its tradition of obedience, has often had the effect of making nurses ashamed of admitting that they felt insecure about performing certain tasks. Group attachment and the extending role of the nurse may mean that health visitors and district nurses are called upon to undertake tasks for which their experience is inadequate or out of date, or which they may never previously have undertaken; these include procedures such as immunisation, ear syringing, venepuncture, electrocardiography and male catheterisation.

There is nothing wrong in extending the role of the nurse for this process has been going on throughout history—the Vincentian sisters used the lancet and the parish nurses of the eighteenth century did the vaccinations—what is important is that extended techniques should not be at the expense of the proper function of the nurse and that *the profession itself* should decide how and when the role of the nurse should be extended. One criterion of the proper role might be the definition offered by Virginia Henderson:

"The unique function of the nurse is to assist the individual, sick or well, in the performance of those activities contributing to health or its recovery (or to peaceful death) that he would have performed unaided had he the necessary strength, will or knowledge. And to do so in such a way as to help him gain independence as rapidly as possible."[5]

If duties are to be extended, nurses must agree that the extension is reasonable and proper safeguards should be taken. The teaching of new techniques and the supervision of the learner should be undertaken by the person most competent to give the instruction, who is often a medical practitioner. Learning from Nelly does not make for safe practice.

Because this subject is the cause of much controversy, the Royal College of Nursing and the British Medical Association have published a leaflet *The Duties and Position of the Nurse*[6] which should be available to all nursing practitioners in both the hospital and the community services.

The safeguards can be summarised as follows:

Techniques outside the scope of routine nursing should only be assigned after consideration of the circumstances and agreement by those concerned. The nurse undertaking the new task should be given proper training and supervision, and should be satisfied that he/she is competent safely to undertake the new duty.

Joint committees should be set up between nursing and medical departments as appropriate in order to provide machinery for reaching agreement on the assignment of tasks.

When a decision has been reached and it has been agreed that a nurse, or group of nurses should be deployed on duties that would normally be considered outside the scope of routine nursing, the fact should be reported to the employing authority and duly minuted.

Although if litigation is being considered, the Health Authority is expected to undertake the defence of its nursing staff, this does not absolve the nurse from personal liability for her own actions.

Because of these implications nurses are urged to belong

to a professional organisation providing individual legal representation.

Delegation

If nursing practice is to be safe, it follows that delegation must be proper. Workers should not be asked to do tasks for which they are not trained or fitted, and no worker should be given a task for whch she was prohibited by legal enactment; for example, an auxiliary should never be allowed the charge of controlled drugs.

The problem of delegation has always been a thorny one in hospitals where there are so many learners to whom tasks have all too often been assigned for which they were not trained or fitted. However, student nurses do bear a measure of professional responsibility, and in the eyes of the law they would probably be judged according to the stage of their training; a third-year nurse would be expected to be more competent than one who has only been in the hospital a few weeks. Until recently this problem hardly impinged on the community health service, but apart from the growing number of learners who now may be attached to the team, the use of ancillary staff is becoming more commonplace and district nurses and health visitors have to consider more carefully what is proper delegation, not only in the passing on of tasks, but in the sharing of information and in communication.

The use of the enrolled nurse in the primary care team has caused some debate. Hockey showed that although the SEN did more basic training than the SRN, there was nothing that the SEN did that was not at some time done by an SRN, the level of responsibility being dictated by expediency.[7] Recently, the Panel of Assessors for District Nurse Training has issued a report on the education and training for SENs which should help to clarify the situation.[8] The primary health care team should be familiar with this report and ensure that enrolled nurse members of the team do have the appropriate training and that work is delegated accordingly. Most Health Authorities have guidelines about the accountability of SENs and their case loads, and all members of the team should know what these are and adhere to them, bearing in mind that although the SEN is a full and valued member of the team the district nurse (SRN/RGN) must take overall responsibility for all nursing matters.

For the health visitor the problem is not so much one of delegation to an ancillary grade, although this may occur in the running of clinics, but one of ensuring adequate coverage during periods of absence. For this the health visitor needs adequate peer and management support and it is important that her nursing officer should have experience in this field. It is significant that in seven of the 11 cases of death from non-accidental injury for which there was a public enquiry during the period 1973–1979 the health visitor in question was away; three were on leave, three were on sick leave and one was undertaking a course.[9]

Communication

The ethical and professional problems presented by difficulties in communication will be dealt with in Chapter 5; here communication is considered from the point of view of what is required to ensure safe practice within the law.

Communication must be proper; that is to say it must be made to the right person, at the right time and in the right form. Health visitors are particularly vulnerable in this respect particularly when dealing with such things as wife battering and teenage pregnancies. Communication to the wrong person can be construed as damaging a reputation and bring an action for damages.

It is important that the communication is understood. The telephone as a means of conveying vital information is a potential source of danger; if treatment is ordered over the telephone it should be written down and read back to the sender; if drugs are involved they should be written on the appropriate card and signed as soon as is reasonably possible. Only in an emergency should messages about controlled drugs be given over the telephone.

Deaths have occurred because patients have not understood the information or message, and claims for damages have been brought because the patient has alleged that he was given the wrong information. It is therefore important that the giver of information obtains a feedback and is sure that the message is understood. The case studies in such reports as *Home from Hospital* show that the records of doctors and nurses in this respect leave room for improvement.

Record Keeping

Accurate and proper record keeping is an important adjunct to safe practice. Records are necessary to:

> ensure continuity of practice;
> give a means of communication between members of the professional care team;
> provide a means of monitoring the efficiency of the service;
> provide information for research into patient care, the use of equipment or the use of the service; and
> give information for legal purposes.

Records should be clear, honest and factual and compiled as soon as possible. Confidentiality will be discussed in Chapter 5. From the legal point of view it must be remembered that claims for negligence may be brought long after the event because of sequelae that were unforeseen at the time. A good example is thalidomide: when it was given to antenatal mothers no one dreamed it could damage the foetus, and the terrible results were not manifest for some time; when claims were eventually made it was obviously vital that accurate records were in existence. The same has been the case when patients have claimed on behalf of children who have, it was alleged, suffered brain damage on account of vaccines. Not all claims are justified and a good nursing record has been a means of establishing that there was no negligence. It follows, of course, that records should not be destroyed.

The nursing team, in hospital or in the community, may be required to keep other records for local or national research. These may consist of statistical information about the patients or clients nursed or visited, with the information required depending on the nature of the research. The team must be assured of the bona fides of the research in question and information must only be given to properly authorised persons. Personal information about patients should never be given without the patients' consent.

In the community, nurses and health visitors will be required to keep personal records including details about the hours worked, times of the week, mileage travelled and by what method; accuracy is of paramount importance because professional people are in a position of trust in such matters and their signature is their word. To abuse such a trust is to bring opprobrium on the profession and, as has happened, cause agitation that the privilege be removed.

Finally, a note should be added about nursing care plans made in connection with the nursing process. Where possible these should be discussed with the patient and other carers and they should not be confused with medical records or the information required by the employing authority. For more detailed descriptions of the writing of a nursing history readers are referred to literature on the nursing process (see Suggestions for Further Reading).

Knowledge of the Health and Social Services

All nurses are concerned with giving advice, but this is probably of more significance in the primary health care team. Many patients have a multiplicity of problems some of which will be interrelated with social and economic problems. If the family is to be helped as a unit, and fragmentation of advice avoided, it is important that members of the team should understand the structure and workings of the service. In this respect the health visitor is probably the best 'resource' person, but all members should be able to give at least first-level advice. Failure to give proper advice can lead to hardship. In 1979 the Disabled Income Group reported that "Tens of thousands of disabled people were not claiming benefit either because they did not know their entitlement or because they regarded it as charity".[10] As an example, health visitors or district nurses may come across people suffering from hypothermia because they fear the electricity bill, when in fact they are entitled to a heating supplement.

Apart from the structure of the service and knowing the benefits to which patients are entitled, the primary care team should know at least by name, and preferably by sight, the key workers in the district whose work effects their clients, including, for example, the social worker, the rent officer, the home help organiser, the organiser of 'meals-on-wheels' and the head of the Citizens Advice Bureau, to name but a few. All group practices should have an up to date *Guide to the Social Services* published by the Family Welfare Association and it should be reasonably available for reference in hospitals.

Corporate Responsibility

If it is a hallmark of a profession that 'its body of knowledge is extended by united effort' and that the profession is itself responsible for its own educational programme, it follows that professionals have responsibilities beyond that of being safe practitioners. Bricklayers are usually both skilled and safe. A profession consists of all the qualified practitioners pursuing excellence and to do this there must be a continual pooling of information and a pushing back of the frontiers of knowledge and, to return to Sir Harold Himsworth, "the continual prosecution of research". Only a few will wish or be qualified to undertake official and funded research, but all have a duty to be research minded and to pool information so that each generation stands on the shoulders of the last. In a time of rapid change this cannot be done in isolation. In the community, group attachment should offer an advantage inasmuch as there can be an exchange of knowledge, ideas and journals between different disciplines, and often the group will contain both specialist doctors and nurses who can be used as 'resource' persons. But local interchange of ideas is not enough, it is important for all nursing personnel, whatever their branch of health care, to have the opportunity to participate in meetings and conferences outside their own locality, and that nursing managements should ensure, as far as is within their power, that such facilities are made available.

Professional Education

For historical and sociological reasons, because basic education for nurses has been controlled by a statutory body since 1919 educational needs have been sacrificed to political expediency. Post-basic education has, however, been in the hands of the profession itself and has been freer to develop as a response to the needs expressed by practising nurses who have identified deficiencies and suggested amendments. Unless nurses themselves continue to accept this responsibility, and say what they need by way of preparation, theory and practice will indeed be divorced.

New Duties and Responsibilities

In hospital the question of new duties, particularly in relation to new drugs and techniques such as the giving of epidural anaesthesia and intravenous therapy, are covered by the principle laid down in The Duties and Position of the Nurse. The position in the primary health care team may be a little more complicated. One example is the primary assessment visit where sometimes there is a thin line between assessment and diagnosis. This problem is not new. Long before the term 'primary assessment was coined nurses were observing signs and symptoms and presenting them in such a way as to suggest a medical diagnosis — indeed, in the days of acute fevers this was even more likely than today. But primary assessment does not mean 'medical diagnosis' and with so many patients displaying a variety of symptoms connected with degeneration, 'diagnosis' as such is often irrelevant. The main purpose of the primary visit is to assess the degree of urgency, and provided proper observations are made and the data faithfully recorded, there should be no reason for anxiety. From the legal point of view assessments are only expected to be what a reasonable person, given the qualifications and experience of the nurse in question, would make in that set of circumstances. Assessments are not infallible, and a patient apparently symptomless in the morning may have a coronary occlusion at night. It is perhaps a measure of the increased expectation on the part of the public that they should be shocked at an incident occuring shortly after a visit from a professional adviser.

The Supervision of Drugs

This is more difficult in the community because the drugs are the property of the patient. When mantelpieces were littered with bottles marked 'The Mist' probably containing nothing more lethal than 'mist. pot. cit.' the omitted or wrong dose mattered little. Now the district nurse must be responsible for supervising patients taking powerful drugs, when a wrong dose could have serious consequences. The same can be true of antibiotics for which familiarity has sometimes bred a dangerous contempt.

The lavish prescribing of drugs for use at home highlights the problem of safe storage and the need to educate the public about the dangers of leaving pills and lotions accessible to children and to instil into the patients a healthy respect for following instructions precisely. Fortunately in recent years, the pharm-aceutical industry has made containers more child-proof (and, incidentally, arthritic-hand-proof at the same time), and all medical containers must state what is in them. This improvement has been brought about partly because of the pressure from nurses acting through their professional organisation, and is a good example of professional responsibility in the wider sphere.

There are a number of increasingly difficult problems about drugs in the home. Because the drugs are the property of the patient the nurse may not remove them without the permission of the patient. Strictly speaking, it is illegal for the nurse to fetch controlled drugs for the patient. Fortunately, it is now possible to control pain in terminal illness better than in the past, but this often implies an armoury of powerful analgesics and narcotics such as morphine and diamorphine; these are drugs of addiction, however, and it is important that carers be instructed how to keep them in a safe place, which may require considerable ingenuity. The administration of controlled drugs as defined in the *Misuse of Drugs Act 1971* lays down certain safeguards, and specific rules apply to district nurses. The person administering must be a trained nurse, that is, an SRN,

RGN or SEN, there must be a written and signed prescription and careful records must be kept. The records must include the stock provided, the amount given, the amount left in stock and the signature of the nurse, and most authorities provide a special form for this. Any discrepancy should be reported at once. Difficulties may arise over the disposal of drugs if they are discontinued or if the patient dies, but the nurse should always do her utmost to ensure that unused drugs are safely disposed of, probably by flushing down the lavatory. If possible, the disposal should be witnessed and the record signed.

Apart from the problem of controlled drugs there is that of a multiplicity of drugs, prescribed or otherwise, which may interact with dire effects if taken haphazardly. This is a particular problem with elderly patients, who besides whatever the doctor has ordered may have their own nostrums. Finally, carers should make sure that elderly and confused patients who may be disorientated at night are not left with drugs by their bedside—many an accidental overdose has occurred in this way.

It is quintessential that a professional worker is paid not only for his skill, but for the quality of the decisions he takes. Usually, the greater the decision the higher the pay and the prestige. Nurses, as Miss Nightingale reminded people, are required to be more than just obedient, they are required to use initiative. If a drug is written up with the decimal point displaced, the nurse would be culpable if she did not question it. If a diabetic patient on a prescribed dose of insulin shows signs of hypoglycaemia, the nurse would be at fault if she did not stop or reduce the dose and report it at once to the doctor.

However, decisions in professional matters extend far beyond decisions about prescribed medical treatment; it is coming more and more to concern the independent prescribing of care and of proper counselling. Professional responsibility now means being accountable, not so much for obeying the doctor's orders, but for the quality of nursing care prescribed and carried out in practice.

References

1 Reader W. (1966) *Professional Men*. London: Weidenfeld & Nicolson

2   Carter H. B. (1872) Letter to Lord Beauchamp, September 14, GLRO.HI/ST/NC18Pkt11
3   Speller S. R. (1974) In *Hospital Year Book*. London: Institute of Hospital Administrators
4   International Council of Nurses (1965) *The International Code of Nursing Ethics*. Geneva: ICN
5   Henderson V. (1960, rev. 1969) *Basic Principles of Nursing Care*. Geneva: ICN
6   RCN & BMA (1978) *The Duties and Position of the Nurse. Joint Statement*. London: RCN
7   Hockey L. (1972) *Use and Abuse*. London: Queen's Institute of District Nursing
8   Panel of Assessors for District Nurse Training UK (1980) *Report of the Working Party on the Education and Training in District Nursing for the SEN*. London: DHSS
9   Sharman R. L. (1982) Child death results from non-accidential injury. Inquiry—implications for health visitors. *Nursing Times*, **78**, 244
10 Disabled Income Group (1979) *Annual Report*. London: DIG

Chapter 5

Communication

In spite of the fact that important changes have been brought about by new technology, that modern telecommunications systems enable messages to be transmitted instantaneously through space and micro-electronics make it possible to store, sort and retrieve in a moment vast amounts of information, most communication is still verbal and interpersonal. At this level there are a number of constraints which need to be understood as a background to the specific problems so often encountered by health service workers. A communication involves a two-day process with a sender and a receiver and mistakes in decoding the message between the two may well lead to conflict.[1]

Firstly, the message may be inadequate because the sender may use a restricted code due to innate poor articulation, or to limited education. Conversely, the sender may use an elaborated code which is not understood by the person used to a restricted code, and this may well be the case between the doctor and his patient. The language used affects not only how people communicate but also what they recall. Secondly, reception of the message may be poor because of lack of attention by the person receiving the message, due, perhaps, to congenitally poor powers of concentration, or to the fact that concentration has been affected by pain or anxiety, a factor always possible when communicating with sick and worried patients and their relatives. Thirdly, the message may be confused by other signals —such as other people talking or the radio playing—or its import may be lost because of the way the signals are perceived. The failure to interpret the impending attack on Pearl Harbour in 1941 was largely due to the fact that the signals were embedded in other 'noise' and when they did come they did not support the expected hypothesis. All too often people hear what they expect, or want, to hear.

Apart from these failures, messages may not be understood because there is a dysjunction between the sender and the receiver and in this respect age, sex and culture all play an important part in how the message is encoded and decoded. This is a factor that must be borne in mind by health workers dealing with a multi-racial population.

In interpersonal communication the non-verbal element plays an important role. For example, facial expression is important because it can, all too easily, register disapproval or boredom, and conversely, approval and interest. It is important to notice how people look when they are listening and whether or not there is eye contact. Looking at the person being spoken to directly is usually interpreted as a sign of being sincere, positive and confident, although, of course, inattention can be dissembled. Non-verbal communication such as body signs, hand signs and gestures can vary from culture to culture and health workers would find it profitable to make a study of the non-verbal communications in the different ethnic groups with which they are in contact.

Fortunately, through the work of Jourard[2] and others, more importance is now attached to contact by touch; the clutching of a hand in fear expresses a basic human need and nurses know all too well that in cases when no words are possible the holding of a hand can bring support and comfort. Ideally we would all like to pass Lethewards holding someone's hand.

Good communication is only possible when there are good personal relationships and these depend on the exercise of personal skills which include the right tone of voice, choice of words, control of facial expression, ease of manner, gesture and movement and the wearing of appropriate clothes. But for communication to be effective the eternal personality must be matched by the correct supporting attitudes and a mental awareness of the situation and what is needed by, or due to, the person with whom the relationship is being formed.[3]

Communication Between the Sections of the Health Service

"Much has been spoken and written about this subject, pointing out that the poor communication lines which exist between the staff of hospitals and the staff of the community services . . . but the dearth exists much earlier — whilst the patient is still in hospital.''

Home from Hospital,[4] from which this quotation is taken, is one of a constellation of studies which included Hockey & Buttimore (1970) Hayes (1971) Wilson & Wilson (1971) Cartwright *et al.* (1973) Hunt (1974) and Roberts (1975), all of which pointed to a failure when patients were transferred from hospitals to the community service, or in the opposite direction. As these studies referred to the situation before the 1974 reorganisation it was concluded that some of the failure was attributable to the tripartite structure, and the fact that the arms of the service belonged to different and separately financed organisations. Now the services have been 'unified' inasmuch as the hospital and the community health services are responsible to the same employing authority, but putting the hospital and community staff on the same payroll does not of itself create a unified service nor yet necessarily good communication.

Many communication problems continue to exist, for although there have been obvious improvements in some areas these have been negated to some extent by the insecurity and confusion that has been created by constant change and the lengthened lines of communication that followed the 1974 reorganisation. The cure had side effects almost as bad as the primary disease. Moreover, reorganisation did nothing to alleviate the divorce between health and welfare and the other local authority services mentioned in Chapter 2, and many advances have been cancelled out by the fact that the users of the service expect more information. Much running needs to be done in order to stay in the same place.

Has the abolition of the tripartite structure improved communication when patients are transferred from one section of the service to another, and has this resulted in a better flow of nursing information about transferred patients? A recent study undertaken by Dr Joan Parnell of the University of Surrey has shown that although there has been considerable improvement there are still problems in the communication of nursing information between the groups of nurses concerned.[5] The study showed that there were wide variations in methods and their effectiveness in different locations, and that little use was made of direct contact and conversation between the nurses directly involved in the care of the patient. Six years after reorganisation 56 per cent of the community nurses said that they received information about their patients, but 46 per cent of the hospital nurses said that they rarely or never received information from the community, and over half of the community nurses themselves admitted that they never sent nursing information to the hospital. However, although communication from the community to the hospital was less frequent than the reverse flow, when it did happen it was usually more complete. This study has important lessons for district nurses and health visitors, who for years have seen themselves as the aggrieved party. It could be that the hospital services have read, marked, learned and inwardly digested the reports referred to earlier better than the community services.

The Problem of Communication in the Health Services

There are a number of reasons why communication in the health services is traditionally poor and why reorganisation has not greatly improved them. It is not that health service workers are more forgetful or secretive than workers in other services but that the historical background is of different groups, with different origins and traditions, working in isolation from one another. The Health Service is still not unified in the way that the Civil Service is where there is a standard administrative procedure throughout the whole service. Bureaucratic machinery may be a subject for television comedy but it is designed to be foolproof and fail-safe, and an official can move from post to post and still requisition on the same form and use the same reporting, filing and recording system in Singapore as he used in London. Not so the Health and Social Services. In spite of computers and attempts at standardisation, District Health Authorities do not have a uniform discharge procedure, nor do they always know whether family practitioners are running antenatal clinics or have social workers attached. The Health Service was not a revolution, but a taking over of the services as they had evolved by 1948. Each hospital and authority struggled to maintain its own individuality and some, like the more prestigious Board of Governor hospitals manifestly won the struggle. After 40 years, admission and discharge procedures vary from hospital to hospital and from consultant to consultant, and while there may be some justification in the contention that standardisation would be inimical to good practice, colourful variation does not help communication.

The other great problem of the Health Services as compared with the Civil Service is that its professionals are trained, or educated, to prepare them for work in different and demanding disciplines. Practitioners must keep pace with ever-expanding knowledge and technical development, and with increasing specialisation it is difficult for one professional practitioner to maintain an understanding of the needs of the service as a whole. Each specialist sees the service through his own microscope, or other expensive 'scope', but the specialists are the big spenders and therefore they have a considerable say in the running of the service.

The administrators, unlike their colleagues in the Civil Service where, except for specialist advisers, all officers are trained as administrators, not only have to administer and carry out the policy of the government, they also have to balance conflicting claims for money, manpower and other resources within one group and between different specialties.

Communication About Patients and Clients

Hippocrates in his oath (circa 460 BC) swore never to divulge what he saw or heard in his practice deeming that "on such matters we should be silent". It has been a long-standing article of faith among doctors and nurses that information received about patients, or from patients, and their affairs, should be treated as confidential, if for no better reason than the fact that unless the patient is assured of confidentiality he will not tell the practitioner all that is necessary for him to know. If an improper disclosure is made and the patient, or his reputation, suffers harm he may well sue for damages.

However, relationships have become more complicated since the fifth century BC and there are now some exceptions to the confidentiality rule and certain moral limitations. Firstly, there is the compulsion of law. The health worker may be subpoenaed as a witness in a court of law and his, or her, medical records open to inspection and there can be no refusal to answer questions about the mental or physical state of the patient unless the judge permits that refusal. However, in actual practice such pressure is seldom exerted. In the case of Hunter v. Mann the Lord Chief Justice ruled "If a doctor is asked in court a question which he finds embarrassing because it involves talking about things he would normally regard as confidential, he can seek protection from the judge and ask if answering is necessary. The judge, by virtue of his overriding discretion to control his court, could tell the doctor that he does not have to answer the question. Whether or not the judge would take that line depends largely on the importance of the potential answer to the issue being tried."[6] There is no evidence to suggest that a nurse appearing in court as a witness has been coerced into breaking confidence, and it is largely up to her to resist improper pressure.

Apart from the requirements of the law there are certain legal requirements to disclose information in the interests of the public as a whole. For example, a hospital treating a patient with venereal disease is required to notify his doctor. Also there is the duty of the doctor, or the nurse, to state that a patient is unfit for certain employment or activity. However, if the patient refuses consent the diagnosis should not be disclosed; an occupational health nurse may well say that a certain patient is 'unfit to drive a vehicle', but unless he gives his consent she should not say that he is subject to epileptic fits.

There is another and more difficult question which arises from the moral dilemma and which is discussed more fully in Chapter 6, and that is whether it is ever right to disclose confidential information to the police to help apprehend a criminal or to prevent public harm. From a legal point of view, a health care worker whose motivation could not be impugned, and who was preventing public peril by disclosure, would generally be safe from actions for defamation and for damages. However, a different view might well be taken if the practitioner disclosed the information merely because he or she thought that it was desirable so to do, a good example being the disclosure to the parents that their teenage daughter was taking a contraceptive pill.[7]

Communication with Colleagues about Patients

While most nurses are quite clear about their duty never to disclose information about their patients to members of the public, difficulties can arise when nurses are told by their patients, or learn for themselves, information that is relevant to the patient's health needs, and which may be vital to other health workers concerned with the case, but they are forbidden by the patient to tell anyone. The question has been highlighted in recent years by the problem of child abuse and other forms of non-accidental injury in the home. Most of the tragedies which have occurred have been due to the reluctance of professionals to share information with their colleagues because they consider that to do so would be a breach of confidence, or if they do so they fear an action for damages. Useful guidelines on confidentiality have been published by the Royal College of Nursing.[8]

If a patient or client begs a nurse or a health visitor, 'to tell no one' in spite of the fact that they or members of the family are in apparent danger, the first duty of the nurse or health visitor is to try to persuade the person concerned to accept help voluntarily, and this can be a delicate and time-consuming task. But not every patient who forbids disclosure really means it, and sometimes the vehement denial of need is really a cry for help. However, there may be occasions when all persuasion fails, and the health worker suspects that the patient means what he says about telling no one, and yet the matter appears urgent. At this point a decision has to be made. In such cases the patient should be told that in his own interest, or that of the family, another person must be told. Generally speaking, qualified privilege exists between colleagues who have some legal or moral responsibility to receive such information. For example, a nurse passing information on to a patient's doctor about suspected alcoholism or malingering would be covered by privilege, although this privilege would be lost if the information was known to be malicious or damaging. If health workers are in any doubt about the line to take on these occasions they may find the Memorandum on Non-Accidental Death in Children, quoted in Chapter 6, useful, especially where suspicions are not strong enough to warrant drastic action. Whatever the reason, the decision to override the duty of confidentiality must never be taken lightly, and the criterion must always be the priority of need. If a child or adult is in danger the fullest information must be disclosed. There are occasions when the price of confidentiality can be too high.

Whether a communication with a colleague is effective may depend on the manner in which it is presented. Fortunately, it is becoming an established practice for the primary health care team to hold regular conferences, and a similar team approach is to be found in other branches of the service, notably the psychiatric field. While this encourages a balanced and a consensus view it must be remembered that some information, or confidences, should only be passed on to the member of the team directly concerned with the patient, and on no occasion should extraneous facts about the patient's private life or financial affairs be discussed. There are some things that nurses learn from their patients that are best forgotten.

Each member of a team has a particular knowledge and should be treated as a peer, except of course where learners are concerned, but learners can often bring a freshness of view and vision that is both stimulating and revealing. It is important that the style of communication, written or verbal, once so beloved of hierarchical and authoritarian regimes, is not used; colleagues should not be told what to do—and ordered to do it—but rather their advice and suggestions should be sought after all the facts of the case have been given. Particular care should be taken with written messages, especially to those whose linguistic code may not be the same, bearing in mind that the dysjunction between the sender and the receiver may effect the way the message is interpreted. In practical terms it might be a good idea to apply the Kantian dictum before putting an irritated pen to paper in a premptory message, "Would I wish this style to become universal . . . would I like to receive such a message myself?" (see Chapter 6). Even more salutary, ask the question

'Would I like to hear this message read out in court?' Sometimes such messages have been read to the extreme chagrin of the sender and to the shame of the profession in general.

One communication between colleagues that is fraught with danger is the telephone message. If the cases that have come before the General Nursing Council are examined, and many that concern advice by professional organisations, it will be noticed that a number are concerned with mistakes in drug administration due to misunderstanding telephone messages, or the fact that because instructions given over the telephone had not been followed up by a signed confirmation the nurse in question had tended to use the instructions as general guidance for use with similar patients. It cannot be stressed too strongly that as far as possible orders over the telephone should be avoided. Exceptionally, one dose only should be ordered and this should be written up by the doctor as soon as possible. The nurse receiving the message should write it down and read it back slowly to the prescriber. Above all, care must be taken to ensure that what was ordered is actually given, and not an intelligent guess made at an alternative name for a particular drug.[9]

Communication with Patients and Clients

A number of research studies have shown that patients do not understand the information or the instructions given to them[10] or that they suffer more pain because lack of information increases their anxiety.[11] Because of these studies there has been a concious effort to give patients more information and as far as possible to discuss their health problems with them. In this respect the nursing process, when better understood and properly practised, should go some way towards meeting the complaints voice in almost every report from users of the service that the professions are in fact 'a conspiracy against the laity'. Legally speaking, however, although the patient is entitled to know what is the matter with him, and what treatment is proposed for him and the risks that may arise, there is no compulsion upon the adviser to tell him everything: some things may be withheld because of doubts, or because of concern for his peace of mind. Moreover, although it is true to say that treatment, surgical or otherwise, cannot be performed without the consent of the patient, and consent implies that the matter has been properly explained to him, in an emergency, or in unforeseen circumstances, treatment can proceed without the specific consent of the patient.

For reasons outlined at the beginning of this chapter there is still often a failure by patients to understand what they have been told and to appreciate its implications; any nurse living as a citizen in the community and listening to the stories of what the doctor said, or what they said at the hospital, can have no doubts on this score. This is particularly true of the patient discharged from hospital who has to undergo the shock of the transfer from dependence to independence, and who forgets what he has been told and hears what he wants to hear. It is for this reason that communications between the hospital and the community service are so essential and that patients should be followed up, although interestingly enough the health visitors placed this group low on their list of priorities.[12]

Similarly, it is important to be sure that the patient understands the gravity of what has been said to him. In the case of Coles v. Reading, a Mr Coles who had suffered a crush injury to his hand was told by the nurse to go to 'a proper hospital' where he would receive an anti-tetanus injection, but the nurse did not ensure that Mr Coles understood what she said, nor did she put it in writing. Mr Coles died of tetanus.[13] Merely telling a patient is not enough.

Communication is a two-way affair and more attention needs to be given to listening than to telling. While listening to what appears to be an irrelevant stream of words it is often necessary to sense the problem behind the problem. Perspicacity, sagacity and experience will enable the health worker to judge whether the outpouring is serious and the truth, or merely a theraputic exercise. If the latter and the listener provides a catharsis, the time will have been well spent. But what a person is saying is not necessarily what he wants to tell; the stream of abuse about the neighbours by an old person may be a manifestation of loneliness and social withdrawal, or the complaint by a mother about the teachers and the school may well be a rationalisation that little Johnny is a delinquent and out of control. Those dealing with such matters know that it is a good idea when nurses complain about the food they should look for the real cause of unrest elsewhere. 'Don't tell your clients what their problem is, let them tell you' is a good maxim. Given patience the truth, and the real problem, usually comes out: generally speaking, only the pathologically paranoid will keep up pretence forever. But of course the 'truth' will only be as the teller sees it. As Strindberg's student said "It is strange how a story can exist in such different versions"—each of which was a facet of the truth.[14]

People ask for advice but most of the time they intend to take only that which coincides with their own wishes. In the last resort, people cannot be advised on personal matters they can only be led to answering their own questions. What counsellors can do is to clarify the questions the person needs to ask, for knowing the right question to ask is often more important than getting the right answer. 'Personal problems' are seldom solved —they are merely lived with with some degree of acceptance.

Nurses and health visitors are in a privileged position to receive confidences: they come as friends, but to justify their positions of trust they must be honest and truthful. The plea of 'tell me the truth nurse' should never be met with a lie, if for no better reason than it will eventually be found out and trust will be destroyed. However, as T.S. Eliot wrote, "Humanity cannot bear very much reality"[15] and it is a wise nurse who knows how much reality patients can bear, and when and how they can bear it. It is a presumption to assume that people cannot accept death and nurses should beware of projecting their own fears and embarrassments about terminal illness on to patients and their relatives. No one knows until tested by adversity what strengths they have, and older people who have lost their contemporaries often develop a philosophy not understood by the young, nor should anyone underestimate the importance of spiritual support.

Communication about Colleagues

In hospitals there is usually a recognised procedure for the appraisal of and reporting on staff, and over the years the system has been considerably refined. Usually the person with structural authority has a duty to supervise, advise and report on the staff in the group over which he has authority. In a team or a peer group, practitioners work more or less independently, although in theory they are responsible to a nursing officer, in practice the officer has little opportunity to supervise and assess the day-to-day performance — a problem that applies to doctors as well as to nurses. Difficulties may arise when a member of the team notices that a colleague is failing in some way; the failure may be due to poor mental or physical health, personal or domestic anxiety, or the inability to keep up with the changing demands of the job. Insecurity may manifest itself in many ways, retreat into sickness, absenteeism, lethargy or aggression, while on other occasions incipient ill health may lead to turbulent relationships with colleagues and clients.

Recently the profession has been made more aware of the magnitude of this problem, referred to at some length in the first edition of this book. Pyne has pointed to the number of cases coming before the disciplinary committees that are due to sickness or personal anxieties that should have been dealt with at an earlier stage.[8] *The Nurses, Midwives and Health Visitors Act 1979* allows the National Boards to

"Carry out investigations of alleged misconduct with a view to proceedings before the Central Council."

This means that there could be a preliminary assessment, and further, that a person may be removed from the Register "for misconduct or *otherwise*" which allows the Council to protect the public without necessarily branding a person as "guilty of misconduct". There is now pressure to have such cases heard by a special committee which has the power to suspend the practitioner pending treatment.

Dealing with a colleague who has, or is becoming, unfit for the job is a delicate matter, but to shirk the issue neither helps the colleague nor the service. There is a moral duty for someone to take action, and again it is a question of estimating the greater good; doctors in failing mental or physical health have been the cause of tragedy because their colleagues 'did not want to be involved'. Failing nurses could cause similar disaster because with the extended role of the nurse and more powerful drugs the nurse's capacity for harm is becoming greater.

Probably the best person to take action is the one most closely associated with the practitioner who is in difficulty and is falling below an acceptable standard. First she should approach the colleague in question to see if there is anything practical that can be done to help. As a profession nurses are sometimes better at finding out the needs of their patients than they are of their colleagues and there are times when a little straightforward practical help would avert a real problem; for example, a loan or a gift from a welfare organisation. In many of the cases that come before the disciplinary committees the nurse has a long history of personal illness, and a background of domestic worry and anxiety, which might have been alleviated before the situation came to crisis point.

However, there are times when it is obvious that the problem is beyond help that can be given by colleagues, and then someone must tell the ailing nurse that, for her own sake, the matter must be reported to the nursing officer. Honesty in dealing with a colleague is as important as honesty in dealing with a patient. Provided the report is made without malice, and to the person properly entitled to receive it and to no one else, it will be covered by privilege. A report if it is true is not actionable, nor is it actionable if it is made in good faith and is fair comment. However, privilege is lost if the report is made, or the information passed on, to people who are not properly interested. So while it would be proper to pass on one's fears that a colleague is under the influence of drugs to the nursing officer to whom she is responsible, it would be improper to pass on one's fears to other members of the peer group, however tempting that might be. It must also be remembered that no approach can be made to a colleague's medical adviser without her express permission and she herself must be persuaded to seek medical aid.

The incidence of sickness and of sub-standard health causing poor work performance is sufficiently high in nursing to call into question whether the Occupational Health Service provided for health workers themselves is as good as it should be. If it is not then it is part of our professional responsibility to agitate for improvements and safeguards.

Data-processed Information

Of increasing concern to the medical and nursing profession is the amount of personal data that can now be stored by micro-electronics and the potential use to which such information can be put. Although protective legislation is pending, Great Britain is out of step with the protection afforded by other European and Scandinavian countries, and is likely to remain so. Considerable concern has been expressed by Civil Rights organisations and other groups that medical records can be made available to other agencies including, for example, the police, and it is part of the professional responsibility of nurses and doctors to ensure that the information that they obtain from patients which is given to them in trust is never betrayed, neither by word of mouth, nor yet on a computer print out.

References

1 Laing R. D. (1965) *The Divided Self.* Harmondsworth: Penguin Books
2 Jourard S. M. (1966) An exploratory study of body accessibility. *Br. J. Soc. Clin. Psychol.*, 5, 221–231
3 Mackenzie N. (1972) *The Professional Ethic and the Hospital Service.* London: English Unversities Press
4 Skeet M. (1970) *Home from Hospital.* London: Macmillan
5 Parnell J. (1982) Continuity and communication. *Nursing Times*, **78**(13), occasional paper
6 Law Report (1974) *The Times*, February 9. London, quoted Whincup—vide infra
7 Whincup M. H. (1978) *Legal Aspects of Medical and Nursing Services.* Beckenham: Ravenswood Press
8 Royal College of Nursing (1980) *Guidelines on Confidentiality in Nursing.* London: RCN
9 Pyne R. (1981) *Professional Discipline in Nursing: Theory and Practice.* Oxford: Blackwell Scientific Publications
10 Skeet M. (1970) Op cit, and Hockey L. (1968) *Care in the Balance.* London: Queen's Institute of District Nursing
11 Hayward J. (1975) *A Prescription Against Pain.* London: RCN

12 Wiseman J. (1982) Health visiting: what will be its function in the future? *Nursing Times*, **78**(18), occasional paper
13 RCN Files (1962/3) Western Area Office. Also quoted in *The Times* (1963) Law Report, January 3
14 Strindberg J. A. (1907) *The Ghost Sonata, Act I*. Trans. Meyer. London: Eyre Methuen
15 Eliot T. S. (1955) *The Four Quartets—Burnt Norton*. London: Faber & Faber

Chapter 6

Areas of Conflict

'. . . and grant that they both perceive and know what things they ought
to do, and also may have grace and power faithfully to fulfil the same.'
Collect, The First Sunday after Epiphany,
The Book of Common Prayer

When Cranmer compiled the Book of Common Prayer
Europe was in the throes of the momentous social change
brought about by the doctrines of the Reformation, the new
learning and the effects of the discoveries of new lands, all of
which added up to a new way of looking at man's position in the
world and his relationship to God. John Donne wrote "the new
philosophy calls all in doubt," and Cranmer himself was by no
means sure what things he ought to do. Today there is a social
revolution taking place which in many ways parallels that of the
sixteenth century; there is high inflation, unemployment, a rise
in the population and a burgeoning of new knowledge, all of
which are ingredients for social unrest. With social unrest and
mobility there is an increased questioning of moral, social and
economic values. In these circumstances men are even more
unsure of 'what things they ought to do'. Any doubt on this
score would be dispelled by listening to a panel of eminent
doctors, lawyers and moral philosophers on the subject of
ethical issues in medicine.

Some philosophers like MacIntyre[1] have argued that moral
concepts like 'good' and 'duty' which had a clear meaning in
close-knit society have no meaning now because there are no
longer well-defined purposes or clear-cut roles in society, and by
trying to reconcile old notions in a situation where their basis has
disappeared, we inherit a 'kind of moral schizophrenia'. But in
fact, ideas of good and duty have survived — although perhaps
in an altered form — through earlier periods when 'clear-cut

93

roles' seem to have disappeared. One example is surely that there could be a 'collective parish duty' for the care of the poor.

Some ethical standards are timeless, for example, the Socratic precept that 'the physician studies only the patient's interest and not his own' and the Hippocratic tradition of 'doing the patient no harm', and such fundamental principles as fairness and the consideration of interests. However, because social customs and cultures change so do attitudes about what is good or the right thing to do, and this is particularly true in sexual matters. Until the nineteenth century most societies accepted without question the concept of arranged marriages — after all the acceptance of parental wishes was enshrined in the command to 'honour thy father and mother' and in 'duty'. The House of Hapsburg and most dynastic traditions were built on child marriages which we now find repugnant. In rural, mediaeval England proof of fertility was usually a prerequisite to formal betrothal — children were needed on the land, and Defoe was not exceptional when he suggested that a child of five years should be able to earn its living. As Professor Peter puts it "Given that the 'consideration of interests' is a fundamental principle of morality and given that there is room for a vast amount of disagreement about what man's interests are, there are nevertheless certain general conditions which are in any man's interest to preserve, however idiosyncratic his view of his interests . . . People are apt to conclude that just because some moral matters are controversial, for instance sexual matters, the whole moral fabric is unstable".[2]

Social customs alter with the emergence of new knowledge, changes in the population profile and new social needs. The social setting has been discussed in Chapter 2 and some of these changes are reflected in changing moral attitudes. The most obvious is that of marriage and childbearing. A society that is facing the prospect of the urban population of the world doubling in the next 20 years[3] and has at its disposal reliable methods of contraception is not likely to have the same attitude to marriage and childbearing as a rural underdeveloped agricultural society. Attitudes to the need for fertility in turn influence the attitudes to women and their place in society. In this respect, in the western world, a profound change has taken place during the past fifty years and it is unlikely that these ideas will be reversed. This is not to say that late-twentieth-century ideas are morally better or worse, they are simply the concomitant of the changed social setting.

Once society ceases to attach so much importance to childbearing and population growth, attitudes to parental rights and duties change, as do attitudes to abortion and, more obliquely, homosexuality. At the same time the growth of knowledge affects what men's interests are. Ethically we are caught in the trap of our own cleverness; rivers of ink have flowed on whether or not severely handicapped babies should be 'saved'. But had not medical science found the means of saving, for example by operating on a baby with a severe spina bifida, this particular moral dilemma would not have arisen. The ethical question now arises, ought medicine to intervene, and if not, why not, and when not? If there are limitations who is to decide what the limitations are? Quis custodiet ipsos custodes?

Allied to the question of the right to be saved is the question of the right to *not* be saved and there is now a tangled web of legal judgements which offer little guidance.

In 1967 the *Abortion Act* allowed that, in certain circumstances, "terminal action against the foetus, and at the behest of the mother and with the concurrence of her medical advisers" was permissible. Then, in 1976, as the result of the thalidomide disaster, the *Congenital Disabilities (Civil Liabilities) Act* allowed a child "a cause of legislation for injuries caused before its birth, provided that the disability was caused by some occurrence that affected either parent before pregnancy, or the mother during pregnancy".[4]

As the result of this Act cases have been brought, but have so far failed, trying to show that a child, disabled by an attack of German measles in the mother, has a claim for 'wrongful entry to life'.

However, perhaps more disturbing to nurses are the apparently conflicting judgements of two recent cases. The first concerned a child suffering from Down's syndrome with an internal blockage which would have been fatal within a few days. The parents took the view that the child should not have the operation and the surgeon agreed. The Local Authority then intervened and made the child a ward of court and in the Court of Appeal decided that the operation should take place because the question the court had to decide was "whether it was in the interests of the child to be allowed to die in the next few weeks, or to have an operation, and if she lives, to be severely handicapped mentally and physically". A question which, of course, defies an answer.

Set against this is the case of the doctor who did allow such a mongoloid child to die and was eventually, after much publicity, found not guilty of murder. Opinions will vary about the rightness of these different decisions, but they offer little guidance, and each practitioner is forced ultimately to rely on his own moral judgement.

More recently, and controversely, a girl aged 13 years, having been placed in the care of the Local Authority, gave birth to a son, but while still in the mother-and-baby unit became pregnant again. The girl, supported by her doctor and the social workers, wanted the pregnancy terminated, but the Authority had the girl made a ward of court so as to place the decision in the hands of a High Court Judge. The High Court ruled, under Section I of the Abortion Act, that the risk to the mother's health and to that of her one-year-old son was greater than if the pregnancy were terminated and they therefore sanctioned abortion.[5] Although within the law this decision was impeccable it aroused a good deal of controversy and protest which indicates that there can be a wide divergence of opinion about man's best interests.

Some of the questions raised by these cases would have been irrelevant a century ago—operation on a frail newborn baby would have been out of the question, and the severely deformed often perished quickly from infection. This is not to say that the past did not have to face the moral dilemma. There was, after all, a choice about leaving Oedipus on the hillside, and Shakespeare's unwanted babies like Perdita who were cast adrift to die were no fables; the 13-year-old in the past would probably have solved her problem by infanticide, the incidence of which was higher than we perhaps care to admit. However, the ability to save life, or prolong it, pales into insignificance as a moral dilemma compared with the possibilities raised by the new knowledge which enables the altering of life by genetic engineering.

ETHICAL PROBLEMS IN THE HEALTH SERVICE

The ethical problems faced by workers in the health service are manifold but for convenience they can be grouped under four main headings. Firstly, there is the range of problems relating to confidentiality and that part of the Hippocratic oath which says "Whatever I see or hear in the lives of men which ought not to be spoken of abroad I will not divulge". Secondly, there are a wide range of problems concerning the possibilities of prolonged life or the withholding of 'the striving to keep alive', and this includes the life of the embryo and life on the machine. Thirdly, there is the question of how to ration scarce resources and who should decide on what, and on whom, money should be spent. Finally, there is the proper use of knowledge and whether truth should be followed wherever it leads, and with this there are the problems of ethics in research.

Confidentiality

Child Abuse

While the legal aspects of confidentiality have been discussed earlier, there remains a number of issues that pose moral rather than legal dilemmas. The most worrying is how to make a decision about the priority of need, and the most frequently discussed in that respect is that of non-accidental injury in children. But while this problem is most likely to make the head lines and attract the censure of the coroner, there are a number of other occasions when the same conflict may arise and which will have to be resolved by the practitioners making an ethical decision. In this respect it is worth quoting the Memorandum on Non-accidental Injury, not only as to what to do when abuse of a child is suspected, but as a broad guide as to how to act in similar situations. However, no guide can help the individual practitioner about the personal decision as to whether to break a patient's or client's confidence, only his own judgement of all the facts can do that.

Memorandum on Non-accidental Injury to Children[6]

(A paraphrase of the main points.)

> Health Authorities are urged to set up Review Committees in conjunction with the appropriate local authority. The committee should collect information, arrange training schemes, conduct enquiries and act as a forum for consultation and consider ways of bringing to public notice the need for cooperation with various agencies.
>
> Staff are urged to be watchful for early signs of child abuse and to take seriously unexplained signs or inadequately explained signs.

First Action

When there is a reasonable suspicion of injury the child should be admitted to hospital, preferably under the care of a paediatrician. Each authority should have a planned procedure for such admissions, and should issue guidelines about obtaining a 'place of safety' order. Parents should be encouraged to accompany the child and stay with him. In an emergency the child should be taken to the accident department.

Where suspicions are not strong enough to warrant removal to hospital the worker should discuss the case with the family doctor and at least one senior colleague in the same profession, or a colleague in a different profession; the risks should be weighed and a conference called.

Managerial Duties

Senior staff should ensure that workers likely to be in contact with the problem have adequate advice and support and precise written instructions. Staff should be aware of the procedure for obtaining a place of safety order and have adequate information about the use of the law to ensure the safety of the child when the parents do not cooperate. There should be a clear statement that major decisions should only be made by individuals in the case of an emergency.

Rehabilitation

The long-term management of cases of child abuse should be kept under review and the course of action to be adopted should be the responsibility of a case conference. In spite of help given by the supporting services there will be times when the child should not be returned to his parents. In these cases departments should be aware of the dangers of receiving a child into voluntary care without a court order or the assumption by the local authority of parental rights. Before the court makes an order the magistrates will need adequate medical and social evidence and it is the responsibility of all workers to keep accurate and careful records. It may be necessary to remind parents of the availability of legal aid.

The phenomenon of cruelty to children is not new; nineteenth century literature is full of references to it, and even in an era when it was regarded as a parental right to wallop a child police records indicate that abuse could fall foul of the law. It is not known whether the size of the problem has increased; statistics, such as they are, depend upon so many variables including public attitudes, vigilance, willingness to report and society's 'labelling'; one group will call it abuse and another discipline. The nineteenth-century headmaster of Eton who said "boys, be pure in heart or I will flog you until you are" would have found the recent ruling by the International Court on corporal punishment very strange. Moreover, some practitioners are unwilling to admit that the problem exists for fear that it will destroy their relationship with their clients; furthermore, although research indicates that child abuse occurs in all social classes, it is the parents in Classes IV and V that figure in most reports, the inference being that the more affluent are better at concealing the facts, and, of course, they are less likely to be suspected.

In spite of considerable research there is no clear guide to which families are most likely to be vulnerable. One study showed that all the parents who abused children had themselves severe emotional problems of a type that would have been manifest to a psychiatrist had they been referred for treatment.[7] On the other hand, the emotional problems of the group did not fit into neat categories. Other observed characteristics have been that insecurity in parents who are themselves uncertain of being loved leads them to put their own needs for love above those of the child and they were apparently incapable of demonstrating love. Such parents have unreal expectations for their children and make unrealistic demands.[8]

Abuse by the family or other carers. Fortunately, the nursing process includes assessment not only of the patient but also of his carers and of noting their strengths and their weaknesses. This is of paramount importance in the community where carers are sometimes tried beyond endurance. An RCN report on the ill treatment of old people in their own homes suggested that in many cases the relatives who were caring had received inadequate counselling and support, and that they were caring for relatives under so much pressure that they themselves were suffering from depression and even actual physical disability.[9]

Apart from being watchful of carers and their stress there remains the problem of violence within the family. This can include wife battering which often presents a problem to the health worker because the abused, and obviously injured wife, often refuses help especially when there are children involved, and unless she seems in real immediate physical danger, it is extremely difficult to take action. On most occasions the best hope is steady counselling and just being available until the wife in question is prepared to make her own decision.

Saving patients from themselves

Recently a coroner complained that social workers and health visitors had not taken action to remove an old man who died in circumstances of wilfull self-neglect.[10] But what right have health workers to take such steps? If coercion is applied in the case of an old man who crawls from chair to sink apparently unwashed and underfed, or the old lady who never goes to bed, where does the coercion end and who decides who is fit to live alone? Society has to choose between the liberty of the subject and the intervention of the State, and apart from rare cases of forcible removal under the emergency regulations of the Mental Health Act, society has chosen freedom.

However, the question of people living alone and unable to care for themselves is distressing and increasing and cannot be shrugged aside. Moreover, with the demographic consequences of the nuclear family, the demise of servants and housekeepers and the disappearance of delivery services of all kinds, more and more old people are likely to be unvisited and thus their social withdrawal exacerbated. The problem applies to all social classes, indeed it is sometimes worse for widows or widowers in Social Class I, who once had household help and are less used to managing alone. The reply of a one time distinguished Brigadier, living alone, coping with his Parkinson's disease and frying his fish fingers, to the comment that "as an old soldier you are pretty self-reliant" was "as an old soldier I had a batman".

The counsel of perfection is to persuade people to accept sheltered accommodation, if it can be found, before their senses fail, and before their mental confusion leads to an inability to appreciate their situation. Perhaps preparation for retirement should include preparing people to plan their retirement in phases, including definite plans for selling up and removal to sheltered accommodation. A few do this already, but even fewer put it in to practice.

Suspicions of Criminal Activity

Apart from suspicions that a life may be in danger there are other limitations on the rule of confidentiality. It sometimes comes to the notice of a nurse that the family she is visiting, or the patient presenting himself at a hospital is, or has been engaged in some criminal activity. S. R. Speller writes: "As regards disclosures about patients and their affairs in answer to police enquiries, which is not generally under compulsion of law, yet may be sufficiently in the public interest to be justifiable, it is recommended that, in case of doubt, the advice of higher authority or the consultant in charge of the case be sought on the particular question involved. Whilst no one would desire, by suppression of evidence, to hamper the police in bringing to justice the perpetrator of a serious crime . . . it is important that the trust of patients/clients in the nurses' discretion should not be forfeited by too ready disclosure in minor matters."[11]

One of the ethical dilemmas posed to a panel of doctors was "A dishevelled patient has left your surgery. You treated him for a graze to the shoulder. You learn of a bank robbery when a gunman escaped with a suspected bullet wound of the shoulder. Do you phone the police?"[12] The consensus view was it was not for the doctor to take action. Whereas, as Speller points out, no one would wish to hamper the police, it is quite another thing to betray a patient's trust and act as an informer. If you start where do you end?

However, there may be occasions when drastic action is necessary. In the case of Tarasoff v. Registrar of the University of California in 1976, the judge ruled that a psychotherapist's revelation of a patient's intention to kill someone "was not a breach of professional ethics since the disclosure was necessary to avert danger to others".[13]

Generally speaking, informing the police about a patient should only be done after consultation with a higher authority and when there is a real threat to the life of the patient or his family, or where there is serious danger to the community. It is conceivable that this latter danger might pose a problem in Northern Ireland: the knowledge that someone was about to plant car bombs should overcome scruples about confidentiality.

Prolonging or Curtailing Life

Does life start with conception or when the foetus is viable? Abortion is a crime at common law, but the *Abortion Act* 1967 provides that abortion is not unlawful so long as certain opinions are obtained, and provided that the termination of pregnancy is carried out by a registered practitioner. It is generally agreed that nursing and medical practitioners may refuse to carry out, or to assist with, a termination of pregnancy if they have a conscientious objection. Although for the most part this clause has operated smoothly there have been local difficulties. An excess of objections in one area may lead to distasteful pressure in another area. However, by and large it is up to the health worker to make his or her individual decision and no pressure should be put on anyone who has a conscientious objection.

Attempts have been made by some nurses to claim 'conscientious objection' against assisting with other treatment they find distasteful, an example being, electro-convulsive therapy. However, there is no real comparison, while a treatment is within the canons of medicine for the purpose of assisting patients to recovery, the nursing practitioner can hardly pick and choose with which treatments she assists, whatever her personal views. Abortion, however medically or socially necessary, can hardly be put in the category of 'treatment'.

Allied to abortion is the whole subject of contraception. Some practitioners will have religious scruples and, clearly, practising Roman Catholics will not work in a family planning clinic. However, the subject is not as simple as an 'either or'; many nurses who would support contraceptive advice to married couples, or to unmarried adults, would object to putting teenage schoolgirls on the pill. The subject raises real ethical problems for school nurses who, although they would do their utmost to counsel school girls against such a course, have to live in the world as it really is, where all too often children have no parental guidance and where the choice is not between chastity and the pill, but pregnancy and the pill. There is no escaping the fact that about 5 000 known pregnancies a year happen to girls still at school. In such situations it is difficult to decide what is the right thing to do, each person must decide for herself; some will keep their own hands clean, others will argue that the prospect of children coping with unwanted pregnancies outweighs their personal scruples. Sadly, the children who are often almost pathologically promiscious, are themselves unwanted children.

The question of medical intervention to save, or not save the life of a severely deformed baby has already been discussed.

However, if the view is taken that medical measures must be taken to save all life, no matter what the circumstances, the same logic must be applied to the other end of life. Is it right to intervene to resuscitate the terminally ill, or to give antibiotics to the frail patient in his nineties who now has pneumonia? Although nurses do not do the prescribing they cannot stand aside from these questions and they can have the courage of their convictions and be the patient's advocate. Often nurses are in a better position than doctors to know whether the relatives are prepared to cope with a severely deformed child, or whether an old person would like to be left to die in peace and with dignity. Whether people advise striving, or otherwise, to keep alive will vary with different motivations and practitioners need to think hard, and objectively, before they make a decision where the overriding consideration should be 'what is best for this particular patient'.

Terminal Care

During the nineteenth century with a death rate of between 20 and 25 per 1000, death, especially to children, was a frequent visitor and was accepted as inevitable and the portal to the life and the world to come. Now, in a largely secular society with the deathrate below 12 per 1000, death has tended to become a taboo subject, and the failure to be able to talk about death is at the root of some of the problems nurses face when thinking about what is best for patients in their terminal illness. In spite of a now considerable body of literature on the subject, research indicates that there is still an unwillingness among medical practitioners and nurses to tell patients the truth about their illness.[14] With the proviso that every case must be judged on its merits, it is the experience of hospice staff that patients should be given every opportunity to discuss their illness with their advisers and they should not be told untruths.[15] However, there are times when the answer to 'Am I going to die?' is rightly eliptical. On the other hand, unless there is some strong contra-indication, relatives should be given as much information as possible, bearing in mind that if the patient has not been told the truth a terrible strain is being imposed on the relatives.

The patient's wishes about his terminal care should be respected. No one is obliged to accept treatment even if refusal means an earlier death, and there is no moral, or legal, obligation to use drugs, or to give treatment, if it is merely prolonging the process of dying.

In hospital, nurses and doctors can usually look for guidance from the Ethical Committee on this score, but in the community health services any doubts should be discussed at a case conference. In the last analysis, if health workers have anxieties about their legal position they can consult their professional organisation.

How patients and their relatives face death may well depend on their religious or philosophical beliefs. Whatever these are, professional carers should do everything to ensure that the patient's wishes are respected and that he is allowed to express them, and that the patient gets the spiritual help and support he wishes to have. On the other hand, patients must be protected from undue influence, and it goes without saying, that professional carers should never allow their own beliefs to intrude. However, when there is harmony of belief there may well be an unspoken bond and support between the dying person and his carer: if harmony is there it should be fostered and valued.

The Use of Resources

At present there are no reliable tools with which to measure the effectiveness of health care. The common measuring rods are the perinatal rate, the infant mortality rate and the morbidity rates of such scourges as bronchites, infectious diseases and rheumatism; but these are not measures of the quality of the services, but more likely, of failures in the social and economic systems. There is evidence that neither the ratio of doctors nor the number of hospital beds has any effect on these figures,[16] therefore the answer must lie outside mechanistic medicine. The Black Report showed that the chances of a pregnancy ending in a dead baby are twice as high for the wife of a man in social class V as for the wife of a professional man and that other inequalities in health also relate to class.[17] Interestingly enough, high mortality and morbidity rates still exist in the same geographical areas and in the same social classes that Edwin Chadwick pinpointed 130 years ago. It should therefore be of some moral concern to workers in the health service that after 45 years of a 'National' service little headway has been made in removing these inequalities.

Although the reasons for the high rate of ill health in social class V are outside the provisions of the health service, there is still room to question whether the balance of resource within the health service is correct. Eighty per cent of the health service budget is spent on secondary care and only 20 per cent on primary care, but 80 per cent of health care is given outside the hospital service. Is the allocation of resource right between the regions of the country, between the hospital sector and the community, and within the hospital services do some specialties have more than their fair share and, how do those who plan the allocation of resource decide what is a 'fair share'? This is not only a financial problem, it is an ethical question. If there are not enough resources to provide kidney transplants or haemodialysis for all who need them, some patients must be selected out; in other words, a decision has to be made about which patients can have their lives prolonged.

Perhaps more important is the question of whether resources shall be spent on prolonging life with ever more costly surgery at the expense of money for the services which would add to the quality of life for those already handicapped. Today, the health service is mainly about non-curable complaints and intervention and support, and this being so, it is reasonable that the users of the service should have some say as to where they most want that intervention and support. The question must be asked, how ethical is it to spend large sums of the taxpayer's money on intervention that can only help a few, even if doing so may well push back the frontiers of knowledge and eventually prolong more lives? There is no easy answer. But health workers who see hardship where there are not enough resources for the elderly, the sick and the handicapped 'who are pushed to the margins of society', must take part in this debate and act as advocates for the users of the service who have no voice, and whose needs are not immediately interesting to medical science.

The Proper Use of Knowledge

Research

The ethics of nursing research must be consistent with the ethics of nursing practice and research must do the patient or subject no physical or mental harm.[18] The researcher is responsible for ensuring that the knowledge being sought is not already available and the object of the study is explained to those being subjected to it, or if this is not possible, as in the case of a child, there must be understanding by the parents or guardians. If for some reason the study is dependent on the subjects not knowing the reason for it, why they cannot be told must be explained to them and an account given when the study is completed. Above all, subjects must be reassured that their confidentiality will be respected. Bearing in mind that a breach of confidentiality in which the subject claimed to have suffered harm, could lead to a legal action, researchers are well advised to have the approval of the Ethical Committee of the body promoting the research before they start interviewing or issuing questionnaires. The exhortation for nursing to be research-minded does not mean that anyone can undertake research. Researchers need to be trained.

Following Truth

Generally speaking, medical and nursing research is not justified if there is no problem, or if the question posed is purely academic and there can be no possible profitable outcome from the study. However, from the ethical point of view, in the last half century, there has been a more frightening moral dilemma, which is should truth be followed wherever it leads? The abyss was first seen by those who researched nuclear fission, some drew back in horror from the prospect of discovering the means of universal destruction. Today there are a number of possibilities on the biomedical horizon such as cloning, or sperm banks to breed a 'super' race, that give cause for pause to ask: should we push back the frontiers of our knowledge if it means opening Pandora's box?

George Steiner, in the first Bronowski lectures, reminded his audience that Thrales, the Greek mathematician, fell down a well while gazing at an eclipse. Looking at the stars he could not see the ground beneath his feet. Men must be free to fall down wells while searching for the truth, even if what they discover disturbs the received wisdom of the day. Galileo's discoveries disturbed the narrow theology of the day, but the truth, and theology survived. No truth should be suppressed, but in the last analysis man has free will to choose what use, if any, he intends to make of the knowledge he has discovered.

MAKING ETHICAL DECISIONS

How do people seek to attain what the Church so delightfully calls "a right judgement in all things"? For many people, of course, their religious creed and faith gives them the basic guide for their daily actions. Moreover, as Piaget has shown, children learn to replace prohibition and constraint by cooperation in such things as truthfulness and not stealing because reasons can be given and truthfulness can be seen to be mutually beneficial.[12] Furthermore, at a number of points the law and Judaeo-Christian principles coincide — what is the right thing to do is also the lawful thing to do. However, the broad tenets of religious teaching can be equivocal when translated into a guide to the social issues of another age, for example, a world facing over-population, and whether total war can ever be justified, and if so when, and for what reason?

In order to help professional practitioners to cope with ethical problems most professional organisations and statutory bodies, including the UKCC,* issue ethical codes, but like religious doctrines these may fail to help with specific dilemmas. The International Council of Nurses Code for Nurses states that nurses believe in the essential freedoms and the preservation of human life and that their actions will be unrestricted by considerations of nationality, race, colour, politics or social status. Does 'life' mean the embryo from conception and include life on the machine? What is meant by 'essential freedoms' — does this mean equal opportunities for health care? If so, many nations are falling short of this freedom. The Royal College of Nursing in its

*The UKCC published its Code of Professional Conduct just as this edition of *Professional Responsibility* went to press. This Code is included at the end of the book, together with those of the RCN and ICN.

document states, inter alia, that nurses should "defend and actively pursue those moral values to which their profession is committed, namely individual autonomy, parity of treatment and the pursuit of health. In some circumstances this may require protest against, and opposition to, social and political conditions which are detrimental to human wellbeing, and in others, the altering of personal habits which set a poor example in health care. In other respects nurses have the right to regulate their own lifes according to their own standards of morality provided that their style of life does not cast doubts on the integrity and trustworthiness of their profession".[19]

The British Medical Association issues a fairly comprehensive handbook, but here again, such general precepts do not help the individual practitioner facing the dilemma of whether or not to report a patient who is suspected of abusing a child. The Royal Colleges have issued the British Code of Practice on the diagnosis of death, but this does not help the surgeon in the moment of decision as to whether brain damage is such that it would be better *not* to start artificial ventilation, or how to weigh the worth of two candidates for the same kidney transplant, nor yet the nurse about which patient to resuscitate. Codes are not a substitute for personal integrity and judgement. But if practitioners are to rely on individual integrity and judgement what other guides have they got other than their personal interpretation of the religion or philosophy to which they adhere?

The other ethical tradition in the western world comes from moral philosophy. Nearly 2 000 years ago Socrates asked the abiding question "How ought men to live?" and tried to find the answer through dialectical logic, working out by question and answer what contributes to virtue and what makes a good citizen. Plato wrote down the Socratic teaching and fused it with his own philosophy. Plato held that 'right behaviour' stemmed from a proper balance of the elements within us and that correct harmony lead to goodness; balanced actions were 'disinterested' actions, they were, in fact, 'just' actions, and proper balance was the basis of goodness and of happiness. The Socratic-Platonic tradition emphasised that man was wicked, or did the wrong thing, because of ignorance and that virtue must be pursued through knowledge. Aristotle, whose Nichomachean Ethics were the keystone of mediaeval philosophy, stressed that good could only be achieved by contemplation and the rational principle, it is this Aristotlean 'rational principle that is the basis for much of the Freudian and Piagetian debate about the ways of developing rational morality in child rearing. The ethics of Aristotle dovetailed with the Christian tradition and more or less governed all moral philosophy until the coming of modern science.

The rational principle took a new line with the philosophers of the Enlightenment who challenged the idea of an innate conscience, and whose work gave rise to the principles of utilitarianism, so beloved by nineteenth-century legislators, and so misunderstood by later interpreters. It was this 'greatest good for the greatest number' principle that lay behind the Benthamite Poor Law amendment and which, for better or for worse, made it possible to force through sanitary legislation against the wishes of so many, and which caused such heart-searching in 'liberal' breasts.

However, the greatest influence on modern moral philosophy has undoubtedly been Immanuel Kant, who maintained that goodness was not an innate characteristic, and that 'good' feelings, like sympathy, often led to wrong actions. For Kant, human action is only good action when it is done for the sake of duty—although Kant never suggested that 'duty' was necessarily disagreeable, it was simply an action that was 'disinterested'—and here Kant is in line with Plato. To find a governing principle Kant posited two imperatives and it is the second that has become known as Kant's Categorical Imperative: "*Act only on that maxim through which at the same time you can will it would become a universal law*". Although much Kantian philosophy is difficult and involved, he does provide a working guide by which to measure dealings with patients and colleagues. Like Plato and the philosophers of the Enlightenment such as Locke and Hume, Kant is explicit about the danger of inflicting harm in order to achieve apparently just ends, Kant is, however, unhelpful about whether war, revolution or civil obedience can ever be justified. Moral philosophy does not provide all the answers.

The importance of Kant is that he brought to an end the attempt to make philosophy a natural science within the traditions of rationalism and empiricism. The questions he asked were not concerned with deductive reasoning and matters that could be answered by the sciences, but rather with the most general and pervasive concepts that concern mankind.

Since Kant, philosophers have tried to look at moral questions afresh and in the light of the contemporary problems, such as how ought men to live in a modern industrial society and how can the principles of 'fairness' and 'justice' be applied in a market economy and whether the ethic of a 'just war' can be applied with modern weapons for universal destruction, and whether, in fact, moral questions about 'duty' can be asked in a society where roles are no longer clear cut.

In the last analysis the individual has to decide what is the right thing to do; the decision will be more likely to be 'right' if the right questions have been asked. If moral philosophy has not supplied all the answers, it has at least suggested some of the questions.

References

1 MacIntyre A. (1967) *A Short History of Ethics.* London: Routledge & Kegan Paul
2 Peters R. S. (1981) *Moral Development and Moral Education.* London: Allen & Unwin
3 Letter (1982) Referring to the World Health Organisation Report. *The Times*, March 11
4 Law Commission (1974) *Injuries to Unborn Children.* Cmnd 5709. London: HMSO
5 Law Report (1982) In re P. *The Times*, May 14
6 DHSS (1974) *Memorandum on Non-accidental Injury to Children.* London DHSS
7 Howells J. (1974) *Remember Maria.* London: Butterworth
8 Lahiff M. E. (1981) *Hard-to-Help Families.* Chichester: HM + M Publishers/John Wiley & Sons
9 Royal College of Nursing (1976) *Neglect and Ill-treatment of the Elderly at Home.* London: RCN

10 Report (1982) Coroner's inquiry in Norwich. *The Times*, February

11 Speller S. R. (1976) *Law Notes for Nurses*. London: RCN

12 Granada TV (1981) *Questions for the Panel*. May 27

13 Whincup M. H. (1978) *Legal Aspects of Medical and Nursing Services*. Beckenham: Ravenswood Publishers

14 Cartwright A., Hockey L. & Anderson E. (1973) *Life Before Death*. London: Routledge & Kegan Paul

15 Hector W. & Whitfield S. (1982) *Nursing Care for the Dying Patient and his Family*. London: William Heinemann Medical Books

16 Maxwell R. (1974) *Health Care: The Growing Dilemma*. London: McKinsey

17 Black D., Morris J. N., Smith C. & Townsend P. (1980). *Inequality in Health Care: The Report of a Working Group*. London: HMSO

18 Royal College of Nursing (1977) *Ethics Related to Research to Nursing*. London: RCN

19 Royal College of Nursing (1976) *A Code of Professional Conduct — a Discussion Document*. London: RCN

Chapter 7

Labour Relations and the Rights of Professional Practitioners

As this book has mainly been concerned with the responsibilities of health workers towards their clients and patients, it seems appropriate to end with a chapter on the rights of professional practitioners themselves. These can be placed in four main categories, namely; security of employment, safety at work, the right to a fair reward and conditions of service and, finally, to the normal rights of enfranchised citizens.

SECURITY OF EMPLOYMENT

Industrial Relations Act 1971

The 1971 Industrial Relations Act altered the position of the nurse in respect of her employment status, because at last the term 'worker' was defined, and she came within the scope of the Act as: "A person who works under contract of employment or any contract whereby he undertakes to perform work or give services to another party who is not a professional client, of his, or who is in employment under or for the purposes of a government department (otherwise than as a member of the armed services of the Crown or any woman's services administered by the Defence Council)." A note adds that 'worker' includes a person providing general medical services, pharmaceutical services, general dental services or general ophthalmic services.[1]

Although the Industrial Relations Act was ill-fated and industrial legislation became the shuttlecock of party political electioneering, nevertheless many of its original tenets are still enshrined in subsequent legislation which include, inter alia.

113

Contracts of Employment Act (amended 1975)

This Act now requires a contract of employment to contain in writing the names of the parties and the date when the employment began, and further to include:

> the scale of remuneration
> the intervals at which this is paid
> the conditions relating to hours of work
> the terms relating to holidays, holiday pay, incapacity for work, sick pay, pay entitlements for public holidays, entitlement to pension schemes and to a pension
> the grievance and disciplinary procedures.[2]

The act entitles most employees (but not Crown employees which includes National Health Service employees) to a written statement of their rights under the various headings within 13 weeks of starting work. However, generally speaking, authorities in the health service do give contracts that cover these requirements and some, such as sick pay regulations and disciplinary procedures, are laid down by Whitley Council regulations. Management should make the handbooks covering these regulations easily available to workers.

However, it should be stressed that it is a basic rule of English law that a contract does not have to be in writing and contracts made by word of mouth can be held to be valid: this applies to undertakings made by both management and workers.

Trade Union and Labour Relations Act 1974

Under this Act the whole body of labour law was re-enacted or amended.

Employment Protection Act 1975

The Employment Protection Act extended earlier legislation about unfair dismissal and entitlement tribunals to award the reinstatement of a dismissed worker; it reduced to 26 weeks the period of completed service before which a worker could complain of unfair dismissal, and was more explicit about time off for union activities and the right to maternity leave.

The most controversial aspect of the new Act was the part concerning the 'closed shop' regulations. Schedule 1, Para 6, lays down that dismissal is fair:

"Where a union membership agreement is in force, when an employee who is not a member of a specified union, or who refuses to join, or who threatens to resign from such a union, except in the case of someone who genuinely objects on the grounds of religious belief to joining a union, or who has reasonable grounds for refusing to belong to a particular union."[3]

The closed shop argument is very complicated because there are a number of different kinds of 'closed shop'; some, as with seamen or actors are vital to both workers and management. Although the worst abuses were amended in 1980, the European Court of Human Rights, hearing the case of the three railwaymen dismissed in 1976 for refusing to join a union when a closed shop was in force, held that the protection afforded by the 1980 Act was not enough. In most European countries the closed shop is regarded as being illiberal in character and such agreements are generally unenforceable at law, and indeed, action to try to enforce them can itself be illegal.

It is against this background that the 1982 *Employment Bill* is being presented (the Tebbit Bill). This Bill's main provisions relate to trade union immunities and the closed shop, and it exposes unions themselves to legal action if employers become the victims of secondary or political action organised by a union. This could obviously have some significance for strikes in the Health Service. Under this Bill damages can be recovered from the unions institutional funds. Fortunately, the closed shop has never been a serious issue in the health services (although some authorities did attempt it in the 1950s) for the not entirely wholesome reason that there are so many different unions and organisations avidly recruiting.

However, the Employment Protection Act had more positive aspects. Unions and organisations, including those like the Royal College of Nursing and the Royal College of Midwives, who were formerly listed on the Special Register had to apply to a Certification Officer for a certificate to show that they were 'independent'. Now, if management failed to recognise a 'certificated independent union' the organisation in question could ask ACAS to intervene.

The Advisory, Conciliation and Arbitration Service (ACAS)

This was set up by Part 1 of the Employment Protection Act 1975 to give an advisory service with the power to conduct inquiries into disputes and to issue codes of practice. ACAS does not normally intervene unless all efforts to obtain a settlement through the normal channels have failed. Conciliation is undertaken by a full-time, experienced and professional staff, and in the last resort the *Central Arbitration Committee* (CAC) has the ultimate power to enforce the findings of inquiries.

The Rights of Employees

Among the rights of employees covered by the Act, those most likely to be of importance to health service workers are:

Medical suspension. A worker who is suspended from work under statutory regulations by a medical adviser will be entitled to normal pay for up to a maximum of 26 weeks. This, for example, could apply to someone found to be a staphlococcal carrier.

Maternity rights. If a woman cannot work because of pregnancy she must, as far as possible, be offered alternative employment. A worker away having a baby is entitled to return to her job at any time up to 29 weeks after the baby is born provided always that she has notified her intention before finishing work. To claim these rights the employee must have worked with the same employer for two years and must work until 11 weeks before the birth.

Trade union membership (this includes membership of a certificated independent union). An employee must not be victimised for joining a trade union or for taking part in its activities. Moreover, an official of a recognised union is entitled to reasonable time off in order to carry out duties connected with industrial relations where they concern his employer, to have time off to attend union activities and to attend approved training courses. What is 'reasonable' may be, and has been, open to dispute.

The right not to be unfairly dismissed. This was the great change brought about by the Industrial Relations Act 1971. Before 1971 workers in the health service could be, and were, dismissed without a reason being given. Now the employer must show that the reason or reasons for a dismissal are fair and that they fall within the compass of the four main categories which are re-enacted from the 1971 Act in the Employment Protection Act 1975—these categories are as follows:

(i) the worker is not qualified for or capable of doing the work for which he was employed;
(ii) his conduct makes him unfit to do the work;
(iii) he is redundant;
(iv) he cannot perform his work without contravening an enactment of the law.

Incapacity. This usually concerns an employee who has become incapable of doing a job because of mental or physical illness or disability, or simply because he is the wrong person for the job, or unable to pass the necessary qualifying examinations. However, if the worker's incapacity is due to illness then he is entitled to exhaust his sick leave entitlement, whatever that may be, before being asked to leave. If the incapacity was acquired on the job, whether or not there was negligence, the situation is complicated and expert advice should be sought. Never resign without seeking advice.

Misconduct. This is the most frequent reason proffered by employers as grounds for dismissal. Often this turns on disobedience of a lawful order; whether the order was lawful may turn on the terms of the worker's contract. For example, a nurse refusing to change her ward, or the district where she worked, would be in a poor position before a tribunal unless her contract stated that she was employed for a particular place and no other. Other misconduct likely to constitute grounds for dismissal is gross professional negligence, theft, drunkeness on duty, and, as pointed out earlier, any abuse of the privileged relationship with patients is liable not only to be dealt with by the employing authority but also possibly by the professional disciplinary committee. Another reason for dismissal is flagrant absenteeism in the face of warning. In this respect it must be remembered that withdrawal of labour which may cause harm, and which is not 'official' can be, and has been, a ground for dismissal. In these circumstances the absenteeism is not only a breach of contract but also a dereliction of duty.

Redundancy. If the employee's job ceases to exist then dismissal on grounds of redundancy is fair. However, in these circumstances the worker is entitled to redundancy payments. Moreover, if the employer departs from the agreed redundancy selection procedure the worker may have a claim for compensation on grounds of unfair dismissal. The Act also requires that there should be consultation with the unions about selection for redundancy and offers of alternative employment. Redundancy payments are calculated on a sliding scale and relate to the length of service up to a maximum of 20 years. The Redundancy Payment Act does not apply to Crown employees, but separate and slightly more generous provisions are made to employees coming under Whitley Council regulations.

Could not perform his work because of an enactment of law. This applies to workers who may be prevented by law from performing the task their employer requires them to undertake; for example, the lorry driver who has lost his driving licence, the nurse whose name has been removed from the Register cannot be asked to give controlled drugs.

Equality of Treatment in Employment

Equal Pay Act 1975

Equal pay for equal work is a principle enshrined in the Treaty of Rome 1957. In the United Kingdom there was no legislation until 1970 and it did not become effective until 1975, and equal pay is now the concern of the Central Arbitration Committee (see above). The Equal Pay Act set out to eliminate discrimination between men and women in regard to contracts of employment, and other entitlements, by establishing a woman's right to equal treatment when she is employed on work of the same, or broadly the same nature, to that of a man; or that the job, though different, has been given equal value by job evaluation. Further, provision is made for the CAC to have the power to remove discrimination in collective agreements, pay structure and conditions which embrace provisions for men, or for women only.

The Sex Discrimination Act 1975

This Act covers the non-contractual aspects of employment; it is now unlawful on the grounds of sex to treat a woman less favourably than a man, or to treat a married person less favourably than a single person.

The Equal Opportunities Commission

This commission has the duty of promoting equality of opportunity between men and women. 'Equal Pay' is a hollow victory unless women have the same opportunities for education and training for jobs, and for promotion, as men.

The Race Relations Act 1968

This Act makes it unlawful to discriminate against a person on the grounds of colour, race, ethnic or national origin as far as recruitment, terms of employment, training opportunities and promotion are concerned.

The equality and anti-discrimination laws cannot of themselves eliminate prejudice and discrimination; that will only come when education and training opportunities are truly equal, and when women, and minority groups themselves, seek to fulfil their potential rather than their expected role. In this respect medicine and nursing still cling to their traditional images; nurses and midwives are expected to be women, and doctors, especially consultants, are expected to be men. Nursing has at least reversed its image about the nurse as a single woman. To a large extent the success of anti-discrimination is predicated by economic factors. There is evidence from the studies undertaken by the Manpower Services Commission that in the cold climate of unemployment women suffer more than men; few have broken into the traditional male strongholds and even fewer into the most highly-paid and prestigious jobs. It is significant that in the 1982 Birthday Honours there was only one woman in the higher honours and only 140 women altogether in a total of 630 and, even more significantly, only one name that could be identified as belonging to a coloured person.[4]

Rights in Sickness and Injury

These rights are complicated and should be set out in the employee's contract of service.

Sickness

Sick pay schemes are becoming more commonplace, and for workers in the National Health Service these are set out in Whitley Council regulations. There are certain basic principles that are worth repeating because they are sometimes overlooked.

The worker has the right to report sick to his own practitioner, and has the right to expect confidentiality in matters relating to health except in cases of notifiable or prescribed diseases. When injury or ill health are such that it is necessary to limit the activities of an employee at work, for example, in cases of epilepsy, there should be agreed consultation between the worker, the doctor and the employer. Injury or illness are not fair grounds for dismissal except where medical opinion states the employee to be incapable of continuing his work (see reasons for dismissal above).

Industrial Injury

If an injury is sustained at work the employee has a duty to report the injury, to sign the Accident Book and the right to claim industrial injury benefit through the Ministry of Pensions, regardless of where the blame—if any—lies. Nurses who injure their backs when lifting patients should claim industrial injury benfit rather than sickness benefit because in the unfortunate event of long-term disablement it is important that valid, properly documented claims are made at the outset.

If a worker suffers an injury through negligence on the part of management, for example, falling down an unguarded manhole, or an injury while saving a patient in a faulty hoist, the employee in question may have a claim for damages against the management or against the supplier of the equipment in question.

The Code of Practice

This code was originally issued with the Industrial Relations Act 1971; it has since been updated but the basic principles remain the same and continue to offer wise guidelines. Although the code is not legally binding it may be used as admissable evidence in cases coming before tribunals. The code lays down guidance about employment policies, communication and consultation, collective bargaining, employee representation, grievance, dispute and disciplinary procedures. In the National Health Service some of these are covered by Whitley Council regulations which are in line with the principles set out in the code. The steps suggested by the code that should be taken when dealing with misconduct are worth reiterating because they are sometimes omitted, and when they are they can escalate an issue out of all importance. The first step should be an on the spot warning, and if the misdemeanour is serious the warning should be in writing and the person in question counselled. Except in cases of gross misconduct no employee should be dismissed for a first offence. If the misconduct continues there should be a final warning *in writing* and the details of the proposed disciplinary action explained to the worker and, if he wishes, given to his accredited representative. No action should be taken against a shop steward until the circumstances of his case have been discussed with an official of his union.

SAFETY AT WORK

Health and Safety at Work Act 1974

An employee has the right to expect a reasonable standard of safety at work. Apart from the responsibilities imposed by common law, all employers, other than domestic employers, have duties under the *Factories Act* 1961, *Offices, Shops & Railway Premises Act* 1963 and the *Mines and Quarries Act* 1965, and in any case the general obligations of the Health and Safety at Work act 1974. It is this last Act that has the greatest significance for health workers.

In 1972 the Robens Report on *Health and Safety at Work* recommended the simplification of the multitudinous statutes and regulations on safety and pinpointing the basic problem as being that of the apathy of the workers themselves, sought to ensure that workers were more fully involved and consulted. As a result of the report a *Health and Safety Commission*, to be responsible for policy-making, was established and a *Health and Safety Executive* set up to impliment the policies. The Act extended the principle of worker and employee participation at local and national level, and the various safety inspectorates and the Employment Medical Advisory Service (EMAS) were brought together under the Health and Safety Executive.

Under the Act, which now covers hospital work, employing authorities have a duty to provide:

    healthy and safe systems of work;
    safe premises with adequate amenities;
    safe plant, equipment, storage and transportation;
    adequate training of employees and supervision by competent personnel;

full information of the staff about safety measures and a
written and up-to-date safety policy; and
safe access to and egress from the place of work.

The activities of the work must not endanger others. For
example, in hospitals there must be strict control of toxic waste,
ionising radiation and infectious matter. Moreover, there is an
onus on all manufactures to ensure that their products are safe
and properly tested. Employees are required to cooperate to take
reasonable care to avoid injury to themselves and to others.
Since 1978 *Safety Representative and Safety Committee
Regulations* have been issued and independent unions are now
required to appoint safety representatives who should undergo
an approved training and be given time off to do so.

Apart from the fact that hospitals are particularly unsafe
places and working in the health services can damage your
health, nurses and health service workers have a particular duty
to set a good example on safety matters as part of their health
education. Although the Act does not apply to private houses, it
does apply to clinics, health centres, doctor's surgeries and
nursing homes which should be, but sometimes are not, models
for emulation.

It must be remembered also that occupiers of houses do have a
liability under the *Occupier's Liability Act 1957*. As an occupier,
a person owes a duty to his lawful visitors to see that his
premises are safe for the agreed purposes of the visit. In practice
this may mean giving a warning to a visitor about a hazard
known to the occupier but hidden from the visitor, and most
district nurses will have been warned about dogs that 'bark but
do not bite'. If the visit is not lawful generally speaking there is
no liability, and although trespassers will *not* be prosecuted if
they impale themselves on railings unlawfully climbing into
parks or gardens they cannot expect protection from the law.
However, to take unreasonable steps to protect property (except
in the case of special security requirements) by such steps as
electric wiring, or possibly a vicious dog, might well fall foul of
the law because children who might not understand warnings
could well be, and have been, injured.

Patients with Claims for Damages

These may, of course, not always relate to injuries at work but the principles are the same. The purpose of an award for damages is to put the patient back to where he was before the accident occurred, inasmuch as money can ever do this. It is, of course, impossible to calculate the value of a lost eye or the use of a leg, but an attempt has to be made and primarily damages are assessed by reference to past and future net earnings with further amounts for pain and the general loss of the quality of life. An award of damages is 'once for all' and takes no account of future inflation.

Patients with such claims outstanding are almost invariably in an anxiety state and it is well known that such victims do not respond to treatment as well as those with no such claims. Many people have argued that an insurance system that looked at the victim's need, rather than merely concentrating on someone else's fault, might be preferable. Such a scheme is already in practice in New Zealand and was argued for in the Reith Lectures in 1981.[5] Now that claims may be up to £150 000 or more, health service personnel are reminded, if reminder be necessary, of the importance of keeping accurate, legible and readily accessible health records.

THE RIGHT TO FAIR REMUNERATION AND CONDITIONS OF SERVICE

What is fair? Is the pop singer or star footballer worth so much more than a doctor, an actor or a teacher? Why does the judge get a 21 per cent rise when the nurse is only offered 6·4 per cent? What do we mean by 'worth'? — worth to whom and for what? The sooner we accept that by any yardstick life and reward are not fair, and cannot be so, the sooner will much useless frustration be saved. However, such acceptance does not mean that we should not strive to find the fairest system we can.

In a purely laissez faire economy the value of work done was simply what the market would bear, which, for easily available unskilled labour, was very little. In a reaction to this system which exploited the worker, Karl Marx produced his Theory of

Values[6] and communist societies aspired to a system where pay was related to both 'worth' and to need. Since then economists have sought for new and more sophisticated methods of measuring the worth of labour, but job evaluation is not an exact science. A new theory (from America) is that public sector wages should be determined by the 'voluntary quit rate'.[7] If no one quits it can be assumed that for that job there is a concordance with the pay in the private sector. But to where does the nurse quit?

The economies of most western industrial societies are now pluralistic with the government forced to play an ever greater role, no matter what its manifesto or political complexion. In these syncretic systems wages are usually a pragmatic mixture of what the market will bear in the private sector with the public sector linked by 'comparability', and what taxation will stand, and of course, how highly prized are services as related to goods.

In the nineteenth century the older professions, such as the physicians and lawyers, charged the fees the market would pay. When such practitioners became public servants, this was their main bargaining weapon. Nurses, on the other hand, have seldom been independent practitioners and when they were they did not command high fees. This was partly because their skills were not in short supply and nursing was considered as being within the compass of any properly motivated woman, but it was largely because those who gave care were women, and women were traditionally badly paid.

The wages of craftsmen, whether apprentices or journeymen, have always been settled by negotiation. In the Middle Ages the guilds performed this function and in the nineteenth century it was taken over by unions. Towards the end of the century the idea of 'unions' and collective bargaining spread to the lower paid manual and unskilled workers. The unions were organised from the shop floor upwards, and eventually, they were responsible for founding the Labour Party, which is the opposite from what happened in most other countries where the workers first organised political parties and, in due course, organised the workers into unions—usually with one union for each industry. This historical difference accounts for the multiplicity of unions in England, where inter-union rivalry can be an important factor in disputes and in wage negotiations.

Whitley Councils

Because of the various different traditions in nursing and mainly because they were predominately women and therefore non-unionised, there was no national pay scale for nurses until the Second World War when the Rushcliffe and Taylor Committees tried to bring some order to the jungle of pay scales and grades. Since the National Health Service came into being nurses and midwives' pay has been negotiated through the Whitley Council machinery that was set up in 1948 to cover the whole health service.

The General Whitley Council is responsible for the conditions of service that are common to all groups, for example, the disciplinary procedures referred to earlier. The Council, which is made up of management side representatives and a staff side with representatives from each of the ten Whitley functional councils, perforce takes into account the requirements of current industrial relations legislation. The more controversial question of salaries and hours of work are left to the functional councils, which in the case of nurses in the *Nurses and Midwives Whitley Council*. The first negotiations in 1948 started with the traditional low level of nurses' pay, and, like all pay in the pubic sector, nurses' pay had to be related to the economic position of the country and how much could be raised from taxation. Taxation is politically sensitive, and with the National Health Service the government is almost a monopoly employer; therefore, for better, for worse, health service pay comes into the political arena. However, in spite of these difficulties strides have been made, and nursing offers a career structure unthought of thirty years ago. Nor, be it noted, does the private sector show much sign of paying over the National Health Service odds.

A history of pay negotiations in the National Health Service[8] shows that nurses' pay tends to fall behind during periods of 'free collective bargaining' and to catch up during periods of incomes policies when nurses' pay has been looked at by outside bodies, good examples being the *Prices and Incomes Board*, the *Committee of Inquiry into Pay and Related Conditions* (Halsbury) and the *Standing Commission on Pay Comparability* (Clegg). Since much time, energy and the squandering of goodwill is involved in these 'catching up' exercises, there must surely be a better way of ensuring continuing fair pay. 'War should belong to the tragic past' — so should strikes in the health service. One possible suggestion is a permanent Review Body as is the case for doctors and dentists. On a more general level, a number of economists have put forward a plea for a move away from uncontrolled bargaining to what is called 'bargained corporatism', practised in some of the countries of the European Community.

For the present however, health service workers are entitled to the scales and conditions laid down by the Whitley Councils. The Whitley regulations, often the accretions of years of bargaining over small differentials, can be immensely complicated and workers moving from one field of service to another may well need advice.

THE RIGHTS OF PROFESSIONAL WORKERS AS CITIZENS

Professional practitioners have the same franchise rights as other citizens. Provided that they fulfil the necessary qualifications they have the right to stand for election to local government; the Whitley Council regulations make provision for this and for leave for workers called to jury service. Professional practitioners also have the right to belong to a political party and to a pressure group and to take part in their activities. Similarly, they have a right to belong to any religious denomination or voluntary organisation and to work for, or with, such organisations in their free time.

However, a distinction must be maintained between the professional worker as an individual and the worker as an employee of an authority. Sometimes, for example for workers of a local authority, the distinction may be hard to keep clear and a choice must be made. If, and when, a professional worker participates in the work of an outside organisation there must never be a disclosure of anything that is confidential to the professional practice or to the employing authority. It goes without saying that no outside activity should bring odium on the profession in question on the employing authority.

Relations with the Mass Media

Most authorities have a procedure for dealing with press enquiries and this should be known and adhered to; this is particularly important when dealing with police enquiries where the question of confidentiality is at stake, and with loaded questions from the press concerning particular patients. Special care must be taken when caring for victims of some disaster that there is no undue intrusion into private grief.

On the other hand, the professional person is a member of a profession and is entitled to speak at professional or public meetings where the press are present. Provided that the remarks are in good faith, are not a slander and do not disclose professional confidential material, the practitioner has the right to be reported, or misreported, in the press without fear of victimisation. Indeed, any pressure put on an employee on this count would now be deemed unfair practice.

The Press as a Watchdog

There are occasions when professional workers, having failed to get a wrong righted through the proper channels, have in the last resort turned to the press for help. Without press intervention the inquiry into the conditions at Ely Hospital would not have been set up and the Hospital Advisory Service would not have come into being in 1969. But for the persistent campaign in the *Sunday Times* the victims of thalidomide would not have been compensated. The professional worker must decide which press campaigns are responsible and which not. However, in calling in the press to right a wrong there are a number of legal implications and before taking such a step the practitioner should seek professional advice.

It is becoming increasingly commonplace for members of the health team to be approached for interviews by the mass media. Although it is a matter of courtesy to inform the appropriate authority there is generally no reason why permission should be withheld. However, those so approached are well advised to clear the parameters with the would be interviewer and to make sure that they have factual and accurate answers ready. If those with knowledge of the working conditions do not come forward, those without may well do so. Nurses are the first to complain that the mass media presents the wrong image of the nurse, either as a ministering angel in some drama, or on the picket line, and they should therefore not despise opportunities to put the record straight.

Rights and Duties

Each professional practitioner must work out a reconciliation between rights and duties. If, in the pursuit of excellence some limitations on rights have to be accepted, it is part of the price of professional responsibility. Whatever the material reward, or lack of it, part of the reward for professional service comes from public esteem, and that is given not merely for professional competence but for the respect in which the professional practitioner is held as a person.

It would be difficult to improve on Sir Harold Himsworth's concluding remarks in his address on professional obligations:[9]

"More than two thousand years ago a code of conduct was laid down for the medical profession. To the fact that the spirit of this code has been faithfully observed by succeeding generations of medical men we can attribute the public trust we have inherited. But the original code was concerned only with the relations of medical men to the individuals under their care. Today medicine has acquired extensive relations with society in general. Nevertheless, the spirit of the Hippocratic oath is as relevant to medicine as it was two thousand years ago. And what is the essence? It can be given in one sentence: Act always so as to increase trust: that is the first and paramount law of social ethics. In your relationships with individuals act so as to increase trust in your professional skill and your character as a man. In your research act so as to increase trust in scientific integrity. In public relations act so as to increase the confidence of society in your profession."

What is true for medical men—and women, is true also for nursing, and one of the questions that might be asked when querying the right thing to do is, does it promote trust?

References

1 Department of Employment (1972) *A Guide to the Industrial Relations Act*. London: HMSO, p.72
2 Department of Employment. Ibid, p.16
3 *The Employment Protection Act 1975, Schedule 1, Para 6/4*. London: HMSO, Ch. 71
4 Letter (1982) An analysis of the Birthday Honours. *The Times*, June 17
5 Kennedy I. (1981) *Unmasking Medicine*. London: Allen & Unwin
6 Marx K. (1948) *Das Kapital*. London: J. M. Dent, Everyman Library
7 Butt R. (1982) How to call it quits in public pay. *The Times*, June 17
8 Baly M. (1980) *Nursing and Social Change*. London: William Heinemann Medical Books
9 Himsworth H. (1953) Change and permanence in education for medicine. *Lancet*, 11, 789

Further Reading

The Law

Whincup N. H. (1982) *Legal Aspects of Medical and Nursing Services.* Beckenham: Ravenswood Press
Speller S. R. (1976) *Law Notes for Nurses.* London: RCN
Rubenstein R. (1947) *John Citizen and the Law.* London: Pelican Books

Ethics and Moral Philosophy

Peters R. S. (1966) *Ethics and Education.* London: Allen & Unwin
Peters R. S. (1981) *Moral Development and Moral Education.* London: Allen & Unwin
Moore G. E. (1966) *Ethics.* Oxford University Press
Mackenzie N. (1971) *The Professional Ethic.* London: English Universities Press
Paton H. J. (1972) *The Moral Law.* London: Hutchinson University Library
Kant I. (1964) *The Critique of Practical Reason.* London: Longmans Green
Aristotle (1953) *The Ethics of Aristotle.* Trans Thomson J. A. F. Harmondsworth: Penguin Books
British Medical Association (1980) *Handbook of Medical Ethics.* London: BMA

Social Policy

Abel-Smith B. & Townsend P. (1965) *The Poor and the Poorest.* London: G. Bell & Sons

Brown R. G. S. (1978) *The Changing Health Service.* London: Routledge & Kegan Paul

Goffman E. (1970) *Stigma: Notes on the Management of Spoiled Identity.* Harmondsworth: Penguin Books

Townsend P. (1979) *Poverty in the United Kingdom.* Harmondsworth: Penguin Books

Titmuss R. (1968) *Commitment to Welfare.* London: Allen & Unwin

Titmuss R. (1973) *Social Policy: An Introduction.* Eds Abel-Smith B. & Titmuss K. London: Allen & Unwin

Watkin B. (1975) *Documents in the Health and Social Services.* London: Methuen

Lahiff M. E. (1981) *Hard-to-help Families.* Chichester: HM + M Publishers, John Wiley & Sons

Family Welfare Association (1981) *Guide to the Social Services.* London: FWA

Maxwell R. (1974) *Health Care: The Growing Dilemma.* London: McKinsey

The Nursing Process

Baly M. E., Rowbottom B, Clark J. & Chapple M. (1981) *A New Approach to District Nursing.* London: William Heinemann Medical Books

Kratz C. R. (ed) (1979) *The Nursing Process.* London: Bailliere Tindall

Marriner A. (1979) *The Nursing Process.* London: Year Book Medical Publishers

The Development of the Nursing Profession

Abel-Smith B. (1960) *A History of the Nursing Profession.* London: William Heinemann Medical Books

Baly M. E. (1980) *Nursing and Social Change.* London: William Heinemann Medical Books

Stocks M. (1960) *A Hundred Years of District Nursing.* London: Allen & Unwin

Clark J. (1973) *A Family Visitor.* London: RCN

Population Growth

Cipolla C. M. (1972) *The Economic History of World Population.* London: Pelican Books

Labour Relations

Cooper B. M. & Bartlett A. P. (1976) *Industrial Relations — A Study in Conflict.* London: William Heinemann
Baly M. E. (1980) *Nursing and Social Change.* London: William Heinemann Medical Books
Department of Employment (1972) *The Code of Practice.* London: HMSO
Central Office of Information (1975) *Trades Unions.* Pamphlet 128. London: HMSO
McCarthy W. E. (1976) *Making Whitley Work.* London: DHSS

Terminal Care

Copperman H. (1983) *Dying at Home.* Chichester: HM + M/ John Wiley & Sons
Hector W. & Whitfield S. (1982) *Nursing Care for the Dying Patient and the Family.* London: William Heinemann Medical Books

Nursing History

Davies C. (ed) (1980) *Rewriting Nursing History.* London: Croom Helm
Smith F. B. (1982) *Florence Nightingale — Reputation and Power.* London: Croom Helm

Reports

Ministry of Health (1966) *Report of the Committee on Senior Nursing Structure* (Chairman: Sir Brian Salmon). London: HMSO

Royal Commission on the National Health Service (Chairman: Sir Alec Merrison) (1979) *Report*. London: HMSO

Department of Health and Social Security (1979) *Patients First: A Consultative Paper on the Structure and Management of the NHS in England and Wales*. London: HMSO

United Kingdom Central Council for Nursing, Midwifery and Health Visiting

Code of Professional Conduct for Nurses, Midwives and Health Visitors (based on ethical concepts)

(1st Edition)

The registered nurse, midwife or health visitor shall, at all times, act in such manner as to justify public trust and confidence, to uphold and enhance the good standing and reputation of the profession, to serve the public interest and the interests of patients/clients.

In fulfilment of professional responsibility and in the exercise of professional accountability the nurse, midwife or health visitor shall:

1 Comply with the law of any country, state, province or territory in which she works, and have due regard to custom and practice.

2 Be accountable for her practice and take every reasonable opportunity to sustain and improve her knowledge and professional competence.

3 Have regard to the customs, values and spiritual beliefs of patients/clients.

4 Hold in confidence any information obtained through professional attendance on a patient/client. Such information must not be divulged unless judged necessary to discharge her professional responsibilities to the patient/client; normally the consent of the patient/client should be obtained. Exceptionally the professional practitioner may be required by legal process to

divulge information held: she should seek advice before responding.

5   Avoid any abuse of the privileged relationship with patients/clients or the privileged access to their property, residence or workplace.

6   At all times act in such a way as to promote and safeguard the well being and interests of patients/clients for whose care she is professionally accountable and ensure that by no action or omission on her part their condition or safety is placed at risk.

7   Have regard to the environment of care (physical, psychological and social) and to available resources, and make known to the appropriate authority if these endanger safe standards of practice.

8   Accept a responsibility relevant to her professional experience for assisting her peers and subordinates to develop professional competence.

9   Have due regard to the workload of and the pressures on professional colleagues and subordinates and take appropriate action if these are seen to be such as to endanger safe standards of practice.

10   Make known to the appropriate authority any conscientious objection she holds which may be relevant to her professional practice.

11   Refuse to accept any gift, favour or hospitality which might be interpreted as seeking to exert undue influence to obtain preferential treatment.

12   Avoid advertising or signing an advertisement using her professional qualification(s) to encourage the sale of commercial products, or services. Any nurse, midwife or health visitor who wishes to use her professional qualifications to advertise her professional services or to take part in any form of commercial advertising should seek advice at the UKCC offices.

Notes to be read in association with the preceding Code

1   It is expected that the nurse, midwife or health visitor will perform her professional duties in accordance with any nationally approved guidelines or codes of practice, and (provided they do not conflict) in accordance with approved local policies.

2   Where the guidelines, codes or policies are found to be such as to impede the safe and effective performance of those duties, proposals for change should be initiated through the appropriate professional channels.

3   Where, from a professional stance, a law is considered bad or inappropriate it should be challenged through the due processes of democracy. Where a practice is considered unsound it should be challenged through the appropriate professional channels. Such actions would be accepted as proper expressions of professional concern and responsibility.

Notice to all Registered Nurses, Midwives and Health Visitors

This Code of Professional Conduct is issued by the United Kingdom Central Council for Nursing, Midwifery and Health Visiting.

It is issued for the guidance and advice of all registered nurses, midwives and health visitors.

The Code will be reviewed by the Council at least once in each calendar year.

The Council requires that members of the profession recognise it as their responsibility (as well as the Council's) to re-appraise continuously the relevance of the Code to the social and professional context in which nurses, midwives and health visitors must practise.

The Council will welcome suggestions and comments for consideration in its periodic review of the Code of Professional Conduct. Such suggestions and comments should be sent to:

United Kingdom Central Council for Nursing, Midwifery and Health Visiting *(P C and R Division) 23 Portland Place, London W1N 3AF*

Royal College of Nursing of the United Kingdom

Code of Professional Conduct — A Discussion Document*

I Introduction

The profession of nursing has a commitment which is shared with other health care professions to promote optimal standards of health, combat disease and disability and alleviate suffering. A code of professional conduct is required in order to make explicit those moral standards which should guide professional decisions in these matters, and in order to encourage responsible moral decision making throughout the profession. It is recognised that no code can do justice to every individual case and therefore that any set of principles must remain constantly open to discussion both within the nursing profession and outside it.

I The starting point of this code is the recognition that nursing is now a profession in its own right, with all the responsibility which that entails. It shares with other professions — notably medicine and social work — the goal of improving the health prospects of all members of that society which grants it the right to practice. Because ideas about health goals vary from individual to individual, and because nurses have considerable influence (and on occasion power) over patients or clients whose needs and handicap often render them especially vulnerable, a code of conduct is needed to provide guidelines for professional practice. Such a code ought to be continuously developed and refined by sustained discussion among nurses themselves, and by consultation between nurses and those who can speak for other professions and for the general public.

*Reproduced by kind permission of The Royal College of Nursing of the United Kingdom, Henrietta Place, London W1M 0AB.

Codes are never a substitute for personal moral integrity, and they can often be hardened into legal formulae. It must therefore be stressed that the purpose of this code is not to devise grounds for disciplinary proceedings (or any similar purpose), but rather to provide a clear and comprehensive document for further discussion, particularly during periods of professional training.

II   Responsibility to Patients or Clients

The primary responsibility of nurses is to protect and enhance the wellbeing and dignity of each individual person in their care. As members of professional teams nurses should recognise and accept responsibility for the total effects of nursing and medical care on individuals. This responsibility is in no way affected by the type of origin of the person's need or illness or by his age, sex, mental status, social class, ethnic origins, nationality or personal beliefs. Therefore it follows that:

1   Nursing care should be directed towards the preservation, or restoration, as far as is possible, of a person's ability to function normally and independently within his own chosen environment.

*1   As a form of social occupation nursing serves several ends: it provides paid employment to a large section of society; it gives individuals a sense of intellectual achievement and job satisfaction; and it offers congenial and rewarding inter- and intra-professional relationships. But none of these should take precedence over the **primary** end of nursing, which is to enable people to live their own lives as fully and freely as possible by providing professional counsel and care according to particular needs.*

2   Discrimination against particular individuals, for whatever reason, should never be tolerated.

2   Entering the nursing profession involves a commitment to the service of persons, each of whom merits individual respect. At times nurses may have prejudices against patients or clients because they consider that they are largely responsible for their own misfortune or because they cannot feel any sympathy for their particular form of distress. But the adoption of a professional attitude requires that all those who need nursing care should receive it without discrimination. No group of patients or clients should be regarded as unworthy or undeserving of professional concern.

3   During episodes of illness the autonomy of patients should be maintained throughout treatment, restrictions being imposed only when these are demonstrably necessary for their own wellbeing, or for the safety of others; and the active participation of patients in their own treatment should be facilitated by means of open and sensitive communication.

3   Nurses share in responsibility for the effect of the multi-disciplinary treatment methods of modern medicine on personal health and freedom. In particular, the routines of hospitals and health institutions and other organisational structures may unnecessarily remove the dignity and independence of patients, thereby diminishing their overall health prospects. In view of this a fundamental aspect of the nurse's responsibility to the patient can be seen as the maintenance and restoration of personal autonomy. This is principally achieved by skilled nursing care of each individual, with an understanding of the context of his illness or disability and with careful attention being paid to communication with him, especially during periods of anxiety. In this context it should be noted that the best source of information about the patient is usually the patient himself and that regular and relaxed discussions with relatives can increase the nurse's understanding of the patient's circumstances and of possible ways in which he can be helped to achieve an optimal level of living. It is recognised that dealing with violent or potentially violent patients raises particularly difficult problems in relation to restraint and patients' freedom. It is essential that clear guidelines are given to all those who have such patients in their care to ensure that prejudice and mutual fear between patients and staff do not worsen the situation. (See the guidelines offered by the DHSS on the basis of joint advice from the RCN and the Royal College of Psychiatrists — The

Management of Violent or Potentially Violent Hospital Patients. HC(76)11.)

4   Measures which jeopardise the safety of patients, such as unnecessary treatments, hazardous experimental procedures and the withdrawal of professional services during employment disputes, should be actively opposed by the profession as a whole.

4   Actions which betray people's confidence in the professional integrity of nurses diminish the ability of the profession to be of help. For this reason the nursing profession should be clearly seen to be opposed to exploitation of vulnerability, for example: Treatment and Experimentation — inappropriate treatment, risky experimentation or experimentation without proper consent; or Industrial Action — the removal of professional services which put patients at risk.

Although choice of treatments and the initiation of clinical research projects is usually solely a medical responsibility, nurses have the right and the duty to express opinions about the effect of such procedures on the patients under their care. (For instance a nurse may question whether the dignity of a dying patient is being respected by procedures employed to delay death; and the design of an experiment involving discomfort or risk to patients may be questioned by nurses asked to co-operate in the experiment.)

Nurses are entitled to equitable wages and conditions of employment and should be free to enter into appropriate negotiations with their employers. But since seriously ill people are in no position to protect themselves when professional aid is withdrawn, disruption of services by strike action and threats to do so contravene the nurse's commitment to service of patients and should be publicly opposed, whether the action is carried out by nurses or by other professions and occupations involved in health care.

5   Information about patients or clients should be treated with the utmost confidence and respect, and should not be divulged to persons outwith the primary care or treatment team without the person's consent, except in exceptional circumstances.

5   *In unusual circumstances it may be necessary to disclose confidential information for the wellbeing of the patient or others in the nurse's care, but this should never be done without full consultation with relatives and with medical and nursing colleagues; and whenever possible the patient should be told why such a disclosure was felt to be necessary.*

III   Responsibility for Professional Standards

The professional authority of nurses is based upon their training and experience in day to day care of ill persons at home or in hospital; and in the enhancement of positive health in the community at large. All members of the nursing profession have a responsibility to continue to develop their knowledge and skill in these matters.

III   This claim to professional status implies that nurses have particular forms of knowledge and skill in health care which are not shared by other professions and which thereby give them the authority to institute nursing procedures and make decisions and recommendations about correct nursing care.

This claim must be substantiated by the profession as a whole through the establishment of training procedures and the maintenance of competence at all levels within the profession and by continued research into new and improved methods of nursing care.

Individual nurses have the responsibility to be self-critical of their professional performance and to seek to adapt it to changing needs and new techniques of care.

IV   Responsibility to Colleagues

In general, relationships with colleagues in nursing and in other health care professions should be determined according to what will maximise the benefit of those in their care.

IV   The goal of 'whole person treatment' determines how nurses should relate professionally to their fellow nurses and to members of other health care professions. It is assumed that the more there is co-operation and communication between the different people caring for the patient, the more the patient's needs are likely to be understood and catered for. (As noted in the previous section, the patient himself has also a great deal to contribute to such full understanding, as do his relatives.)

1   Professional relationships between nurses should be regulated according to the level of knowledge, experience and skill of each nurse. Clear chains of command should be established to deal with emergency situations, but except in such situations, free discussion of the reasons for established procedures should be encouraged at all levels.

1   The nursing 'hierarchy' can be seen to be necessary to ensure that decisions are taken by those who should have the requisite knowledge and experience, but on the other hand junior members of staff can often bring fresh insights about patients or be more successful in gaining the patient's confidence. For this reason an atmosphere of friendly questioning and discussion between staff at different levels can improve the quality of care as well as making nurse education more effective. (Obviously clear lines of authority are needed for situations in which rapid decisions have to be made.)

2   Professional relationships between nurses and doctors should be regulated according to the particular expertise of each profession. In the case of medical treatments nurses are under an obligation to carry out a doctor's instructions except where they have a good reason to believe that harm will be caused to the patient by so doing. In cases in which nurses' continuous contact with the patient has given them a different insight into the patient's medical needs, they are under moral obligation to communicate this to the doctor in charge of the case. Nurses should support the multi-disciplinary case-conference approach to treatment decisions, and should improve their ability to participate actively in such conferences.

2   Nurses are not trained to diagnose illness or to prescribe medical treatment. They must therefore normally carry out doctors' instructions in these matters and help maintain the patient's confidence in his medical advisers. But nurses are in a unique position to observe the condition of the patient at all hours of day and night and have received basic instruction in drug dosages, effects of treatment, etc. For this reason they are morally obliged to question medical instructions which the believe will cause the patient harm or unnecessary distress, (see Section II) even though they may fear adverse effects on their career from doing so. Ideally, however, this should not entail a confrontation between doctor and nurse, but should arise naturally in the context of ongoing inter-professional discussions in case conferences. Part of the professional training of nurses should prepare them to take part in such conferences from their own professional standpoint.

3 Professional relationships between nurses and members of other health care professions should be based upon respect for each other's area of expertise and on the desire to gain a fuller understanding of the patient's or client's needs. Procedures should be established for regular inter-professional consultations.

3 In the case of other professions which may have contact with patients or clients (e.g. para-medical professions, social workers, hospital chaplains and other clergy) nurses should be concerned to establish relationships of trust. This should promote a mutual understanding of professional roles enabling the patient/client to derive maximum benefit from the work of the caring team.

V Professional Responsibilty and Personal Responsibility

As citizens of a state and as private individuals nurses should defend and actively pursue those moral values to which their profession is committed, namely, individual autonomy, parity of treatment and the pursuit of health. In some circumstances this may require protest against, and opposition to, social and political conditions which are detrimental to human wellbeing; and in others, the altering of personal habits which set a poor example in health care. In all other respects nurses have the right to regulate their private lives according to their own standards of morality, provided their style of life does not cast doubts on the integrity and trustworthiness of their profession.

V Because nursing finds its origins partly in religious orders, there may be unrealistic expectations both within the profession and among the general public about the degree of personal dedication to which modern nurses should aspire. Like other professionals, nurses have the right to conduct their private lives without undue interference from colleagues or employers. Also like other professionals, however, the choice of a personal service career commits the nurse to certain moral views. Nurses cannot strive to alleviate disease and suffering without becoming aware of the social circumstances which bring it about or which inhibit the provision of effective remedies. It follows that nurses should be concerned with political and social issues, whenever these are relevant to the prevention of disease or the delivery of health care. Similarly in the sphere of personal conduct, nurses should strive to 'practise what they preach' to avoid personal habits which are known to be detrimental to health. (For example, doctors and nurses are particularly at risk for drug and alcohol addiction—a factor which seems to demand closer supportive attention from their respective professions.)

In addition to setting a good example in healthy styles of life, nurses need to inspire confidence in patients in order to be able to help them fully. This does not imply 'angelic' purity of life—merely the following of standards of honesty and of moral seriousness which would be expected from any member of society who has responsibility for the welfare of others.

International Council of Nurses

Code for Nurses

Ethical Concepts Applied to Nursing

It was at the meeting of the Grand Council of the International Council of Nurses (ICN) held in Sao Paulo, Brazil, in July 1953, that an international code of ethics for nurses was first adopted. The Grand Council subsequently revised the Code at its meeting in Frankfurt, Germany, in June 1965. The Code for Nurses, reproduced here by kind permission of the International Council of Nurses, was adopted by the ICN Council of National Representatives in Mexico City in May 1973. The Suggestions for Application of the Concepts and Suggestions for Distribution and Use of the Code were produced by the Professional Services Committee of ICN in September 1974. They were prepared and designed to be used in conjunction with the Code for Nurses.

The fundamental responsibility of the nurse is fourfold: to promote health, to prevent illness, to restore health and to alleviate suffering.

The need for nursing is universal. Inherent in nursing is respect for life, dignity and rights of man. It is unrestricted by considerations of nationality, race, creed, colour, age, sex, politics or social status.

Nurses render health services to the individual, the family and the community and coordinate their services with those of related groups.

Nurses and People

The nurse's primary responsibility is to those people who require nursing care.

The nurse, in providing care, promotes an environment in which the values, customs and spiritual beliefs of the individual are respected.

The nurse holds in confidence personal information and uses judgement in sharing this information.

Nurses and Practice

The nurse carries personal responsibility for nursing practice and for maintaining competence by continual learning.

The nurse maintains the highest standards of nursing care possible within the reality of a specific situation.

The nurse uses judgement in relation to individual competence when accepting and delegating responsibilities.

The nurse when acting in a professional capacity should at all times maintain standards of personal conduct which reflect credit upon the profession.

Nurses and Society

The nurse shares with other citizens the responsibility for initiating and supporting action to meet the health and social needs of the public.

Nurses and Co-Workers

The nurse sustains a cooperative relationship with co-workers in nursing and other fields.

The nurse takes appropriate action to safeguard the individual when his care is endangered by a co-worker or any other person.

Nurses and the Profession

The nurse plays the major role in determining and implementing desirable standards of nursing practice and nursing education.

The nurse is active in developing a core of professional knowledge.

The nurse, acting through the professional organisation, participates in establishing and maintaining equitable social and economic working conditions in nursing.

Suggestions for application by nursing educators, practitioners, administrators and nurses' associations of concepts of the Code for Nurses

The *Code for Nurses* is a guide for action based on values and needs of society. It will have meaning only if it becomes a living document applied to the realities of human behaviour in a changing society.

In order to achieve its purpose the *Code* must be understood, internalized and utilized by nurses in all aspects of their work. It must be put before and be continuously available to students and practitioners in their mother tongue, throughout their study and work lives. For practical application in the local setting, the *Code* should be studied in conjunction with information relevant to the specific situation which would guide the nurse in selecting priorities and scope for action in nursing.

These suggestions need to be adapted, expanded and supplemented by additional items.

Headings of the **Code for Nurses**	Educators	Practitioners and administrators	Nurses' associations
NURSES AND PEOPLE	Person-focused education (individual and community) Health-oriented education Study of social and behavioural sciences	Person-focused practice Respect for values, customs and beliefs Comprehensive care System for guarding confidentiality	Acceptance of responsibility in nursing education and practice
NURSES AND PRACTICE	Judgement skills Attitude and skills for continued learning	Support system for nursing judgement Learning opportunities in service situations Organization of service to promote quality care	Legislative safeguards for nursing practice Continuing education programmes Working conditions to ensure continuing education
NURSES AND SOCIETY	Student participation in community experience Citizen involvement in educational programmes	Involvement in community action Consumer participation in health care delivery	Position papers on social issues Cooperation with other professional and social groups
NURSES AND CO-WORKERS	Understanding of role of other workers Communication of role of nursing to other professions	Awareness of specific and overlapping functions System for collaboration	Cooperation with associations of other disciplines
NURSES AND THE PROFESSION	Active membership in association Standards for nursing education Research and communications skills Understanding of nursing as a profession Support of student nurses association	Active membership in association Standards for nursing practice Individual contribution through research publications Cooperation with student nurses association	Large, active membership Guidelines for standards in nursing Research and publications Equitable social and economic status and working conditions through legislative representation and collective bargaining Support of and cooperation with student nurses association

**Suggestions for Distribution
and Use of the Code for Nurses**

Who	Why	How - When - Where
Students and practitioners of nursing	Promotion of professional knowledge, attitudes and behaviour Use of the **Code** in daily practice particularly the key aspects of responsibility and judgement Assessment of professional performance Awareness of possible conflicts between ethical concepts of the **Code** and personal beliefs Basis for legislation affecting nursing Involvement in adapting the **Code** to changing society	All educational programmes Nursing and related press, textbooks and updated bibliography Professional seminars and meetings
Students and practitioners in other fields	Cooperation and coordination between nurses and practitioners in other fields	Educational programmes Specific press and publications Interdisciplinary seminars and meetings
General public	Communication between nurses and the public in relation to nursing and the **Code** Recruitment of candidates for nursing	Mass media Contact with consumer and policy-making groups and other organizations Career counselling

Index